MASTERING MENTALIZATION

MASTERING MENTALIZATION

Taking, Gaining, Shifting and Shaping Perspectives Through Basic, Affective and Strategic Mentalizing

Complete Volume

Anique van der Putten

Edited by Dennis Weyrauch

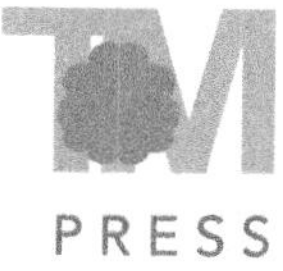

PRESS

Edited by Dennis Weyrauch
Book cover image and book design by Anique van der Putten

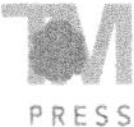

Publisher: ToM PRESS
ToM PRESS is an imprint of the Center for Applied Theory of Mind

First published 2022

Mastering Mentalization: Complete Volume
ISBN: 978-989-53691-1-9 (hardcover)
ISBN: 978-989-53691-0-2 (paperback)

Other Volumes:
Mastering Mentalization: Volume I, Basic Mentalizing
ISBN: 978-989-53691-2-6 (paperback)
Mastering Mentalization: Volume II, Affective Mentalizing
ISBN: 978-989-53691-3-3 (paperback)
Mastering Mentalization: Volume III, Strategic Mentalizing
ISBN: 978-989-53691-4-0 (paperback)

The Mentalization Journal
ISBN: 978-989-53691-5-7 (hardcover)
ISBN: 978-989-53691-6-4 (paperback)

Descriptions of these publications can be found at: www.appliedtom.com

MASTERING MENTALIZATION

Contents

MASTERING MENTALIZATION

Introduction

Over the course of our lives there are many occasions when we wish we could read the minds of others. The good news is, we actually can, although only to a certain extent, and not in a magical or mystical way. The fact that there is nothing mystical in the way we mindread does not mean that it isn't still one of our most fascinating social abilities. This book is designed to arouse your interest in the most powerful social tool at your disposal: Mentalization.

Mentalization pertains to our ability to *take, gain, shift* and *shape* the *perspectives* of others. We use these mentalization abilities as a guide to explain or predict behavior. The mentalization process starts with the detection of social signals and cues in the verbal and nonverbal behavior of others. It continues with the attachment of meaning to these social indicators. These meaningful inferences allow us to explain past behavior and to predict future behavior. Our own perspectives are likewise inferred through a mentalization process.

Mentalization lies at the core of the key cognitive processes that we use to interpret and guide social behavior. It is, by and large, an interpersonal endeavor that we rely upon in order to make social interactions run more smoothly and at the same time achieve our objectives. In addition, we use our mentalization capacities to assess the trustworthiness and competence of others, helping us to make better social affiliation decisions. Mentalization is critical to successful affiliation and cooperation with others. It is also key to gaining competitive advantage over others or socially distancing ourselves from those whose interests do not align with our own. The motivational impetus to mentalize about others is innate. The tendency is so strong, in fact, that we even infer mental states in non-human entities, such as cars or computers, thereby anthropomorphizing them. Mentalization has actually played an important role in the emergence of religious beliefs and devotion to a personified higher power.

Mentalization is a multifaceted concept, which operates on many different layers. Although the constituent components of mentalization are closely interconnected, we have identified three distinct levels of mentalization: *basic, affective* and *strategic.* We call the first level basic mentalizing as it involves the most elementary level of mentalization at which we derive basic mental state inferences by reading nonverbal behaviors and our sensorial reactions to them. Basic mentalizing reveals straightforward goal-directed behavior and primary affective states. The second level is labeled affective mentalizing, as it involves our ability to make more complex affective mental state inferences that help us to regulate emotions, feelings and moods that advance or impede our social interaction and our mentalization efforts. We call the third level strategic mentalizing, as it involves the most cognitive level of mentalization, enabling us to infer the more epistemic (cognitive) mental states such as desire, belief, knowledge and intention. We refer to this level as strategic mentalizing since it involves the prediction or explanation of increasingly complex goal-directed behavior. Strategic mentalizing is an ongoing, iterative and cyclical process that coalesces in a comprehensive theory of mind. This level represents the integration of all three levels of mentalization: basic, affective and strategic. In other words, accurate complex mental state inferences are the result of an iterative process by which we navigate among the three levels of mentalization during our interactions with others. Additionally, strategic mentalizing is an iterative process in the sense that we repeatedly move forward and backward in time to gather and connect social information from events in the past, from the present and from our predictions of possible future scenarios. Accurate mental state inferences are likewise the result of a co-creative, iterative endeavor involving interactional partners.

The complexity of mentalization has attracted the interests of scientists, philosophers and psychologists, as well as others from wide-ranging fields of interest, each with their own distinct perspectives on what mentalization entails, giving rise to the many synonyms for mentalization. To name just a few: "theory of mind" (Premack & Woodruff, 1978), "mind-reading" (Whiten, 1991), "folk psychology" (Gordon, 1986), and "the intentional stance" (Dennett, 1987). Our view of the subject matter is best represented by the verb "mentalize," the noun "mentalization" and the term "theory of mind." The verb "mentalize" was first used by Frith et al. (1991) in their paper on theory of mind in relation to autism. Because mentalization is a behavioral process (i.e., something we do), a verb is well fitting. Mindreading is also a useful verb, although in its colloquial use it has gained a mystical connotation, which tends to conflict with our objective of demystifying both the overall ability and its constituent components. We use the noun "mentalization" to refer to the more general concept of the act of mentalizing. We also decided to adopt the term "theory of mind" when discussing the highest level of mentalization that we refer to as strategic mentalizing. The term was coined by Premack and Woodruff (1978) in their paper entitled "*Does the Chimpanzee Have a Theory of Mind?*" Theory of mind refers to the human capacity to construct and evaluate increasingly rational models of what is going on in the minds of others. It demarks the point at which we step away from common-sense psychology and mentalize on a more abstract level, applying psychological theory to human behavior and reasoning.

Philosophers have played an important role in kindling interest in the subject of mentalization, and later in the development of empirical research on the topic. Descartes' *Second Meditation* (Descartes, 2008), where he discussed "[t]he nature of the human mind, and how it is better known than the body," set the groundwork for considering the science of the mind. He regarded the mental state of knowledge, particularly the capacity to doubt this particular mental state, as evidence of the fact that we exist. His famous adage "*Cogito, ergo sum*" ("I think therefore I am") was born out of the need to defend his views. Within the contemporary branch of philosophy known as "philosophy of mind" two dominant theoretical views emerged to explain how it is that we are able to mentalize. According to one view, "theory theory" (see Gopnik & Wellman, 1994) derived from Morton (1980), we come to an understanding of the minds of others through *the deployment of a theory* that relies upon an understanding of mental state concepts and behavioral laws and principles to explain and predict behavior. In several fundamental aspects, theory theory stands in contrast to a second view known as "simulation theory" (see Harris, 1992; Goldman, 2006; Gordon, 1992).

Simulation theory takes the position that *mentalization may not depend upon a fully specified theory of mind*. Instead, we use our empathic abilities to simulate the minds of others, or we project our own mental states onto the minds of others and assume that they feel and think as we do. The contrasting views represented by these two theories have provided fodder for interesting debates that have advanced scientific understanding of the various components and layers of mentalization. In our opinion, both *theory theory and simulation theory have a proper place within the study of mentalization as basic and affective mentalizing approximate simulation theory, while strategic mentalizing tracks closer to theory theory*.

In the twentieth century mentalization was examined by a field of research known as "belief-desire psychology," also referred to as "folk psychology." For instance, Daniel Dennett (1987 p. 17), an American philosopher, writer and cognitive scientist, proposed the procedure of mentalization as follows:

> Here is how it works: first you decide to treat the object whose behavior is to be predicted as a rational agent; then you figure out what beliefs that agent ought to have, given its place in the world and its purpose. Then you figure out what desires it ought to have, on the same considerations, and finally you predict that this rational agent will act to further its goals in the light of its beliefs. A little practical reasoning from the chosen set of beliefs and desires will in most instances yield a decision about what the agent ought to do; that is what you predict the agent will do.

He referred to this process as "the intentional stance." Dennett's philosophical proposition spawned many insightful debates. Belief-desire psychology does not, however, explain the full extent of what is needed to understand a person's motivations or intentions, which Dennett also recognized by his subsequent inclusion of additional factors. To begin with, because belief-desire psychology *primarily focuses on beliefs and desires,* it ignores a vast range of mental state information that must be taken into account in order to accurately predict or explain complex behavior. For instance, affect and knowledge are two primary mental state categories which, together with desire and belief, make up increasingly complex mental states such as intentions, motivations and attitudes. Additionally, contextual and situational factors, such as social environment, have a significant influence on mental states and behavior. Predictions and explanations of behavior need to be based upon the range of behavioral possibilities for the particular person about whom we are mentalizing. Furthermore, predictions of complex behavior should never be made on the basis of what a person *ought* to do. Many studies have shown that humans often do not follow "logical rules" in their behavioral choices. Predictions and explanations need to be tailored to the individual within context, which requires consideration of all factors of influence. By taking all of these factors into account we are able to evaluate all of the different possible behaviors that the person might choose, and assign probabilities to each. The behavior with the highest probability will generally be our best bet. In other words, we have to predict complex behavior on the basis of what the person in question is *most likely* to do, rather than what the person ought to do. In 1971, Dennett injected the following into his intentional stance proposition: "a personal stance," which not only "presupposes the intentional stance," (viz., treats the system as rational) but also views it as "a person" (Dennett, 1971/1978, p. 240). Here we see the emergence in Dennett's proposition of a more personalized perspective in predicting behavior.

Mentalization has been, and continues to be, extensively studied in connection with the developmental trajectory of children. The vast majority of research to date has focused exclusively on abstract mental state reasoning of children. For instance, many research papers focus on "false-belief" reasoning, which is the ability to reason about another person's beliefs with the understanding that those beliefs can differ from reality, an important aspect of perspective gaining. This strong focus on the development of abstract mental state concepts has given prominence to the theory of mind aspects of mentalization. However, some mentalizing of *non*-propositional mental states, affective mental states in particular, can be done through the use of *common-sense psychology, simulation*, or *projection* as it does not require propositional mental state reasoning to predict or explain behavior.

Research on mentalization has expanded beyond the study of early childhood development. Scholars in the field of artificial intelligence are conducting extensive research into how computers and humanoid robots can be programmed to mentalize about humans. Turing, one of the founders of artificial intelligence, was the first to ask the question "*Can machines think?*" (Turing, 1950). Turing introduced an imitation game, which became known as the "Turing Test," to test whether artificial intelligence can equal human intelligence. This game involves a test subject who communicates through a teleprompter with two agents in another room. One agent is a human being, and the other is a computer. The test subject asks both agents questions and the agents have to answer those questions. When the computer "passes" the Turing Test it means that it has tricked the test person into believing that it is the human. The ability to deceive others by altering their belief state requires insight into their minds. In other words, the ability to mentalize about humans is imperative for computers and humanoid robots to pass the Turing Test. Scientists in the field of "game theory" are particularly interested in the strategic aspects of mentalization. Game theory focuses on interactive decisions where behavioral strategies, either *cooperative* or *competitive*, of two or more people jointly determine an outcome that affects all of them. This field of research also studies strategies of "cheaters." Cheaters often use mentalization to manipulate and deceive others. Researchers in the area of evolution focus on questions such as: Has mentalization developed for *cooperative planning* and to *strengthen social cohesion*, or has it developed principally to *deceive competitors* or to *recognize deception*? To place mentalization in an evolutionary context, scientists primarily use behavioral theories based on research with primates. Humans, however, have distinct capabilities, for instance the use of "language" and "mental time travel" (the capacity to project oneself into scenarios in the past, alternative scenarios in the present, or future scenarios). Do primates mentalize? Results are still inconclusive. Ape-like species such as chimpanzees and bonobos display signs of having a theory of mind, however, this might be more in terms of "perception-goal" inferences than in terms of mentalizing. They might, for example, just look at an object in which another primate shows interest, and predict behavior without consideration of the other's mental state. There are also scholars who study mentalization abilities in nonprimates. The goal of such studies is to determine whether these animals are capable of forming the conceptual understanding of what is going on in another animal's mind, or whether, instead, they learn to predict behavior through perception-goal inferences. For instance, let us say a dog detects sadness in its owner's voice. The dog tries to cheer up its owner by wagging its tail and lavishly licking its owner's hand as an appeasement gesture. Does this mean that the dog infers its owner's mental states of sadness and desire to be consoled (a theory of mind), or does it merely want to lower its own stress level through behavior that dogs instinctively employ when another pack member is in distress (a perception-goal inference)? Attempts to prove the existence of a theory of mind in nonhuman species can be exceedingly complex as researchers are not able to rely on verbal confirmations. Social neuroscientists study the "social information-processing architecture" and "functionality" of mentalization. Neurological research on mentalization shows that the ability to mentalize encompasses a variety of cognitive processes that have been developed at different times, over millions of years, and for a variety of reasons. These processes have had different developmental trajectories. Some neural system elements implicated in mentalization are part of systems that developed earlier in our evolution, while other elements belong to more recently developed neural architectures. Neurological insights, in addition to making it possible to map the neurological architecture and functionality of our mentalization efforts, are also critical to understanding discrepancies in the mentalization abilities of different people. These research outcomes add valuable information to studies conducted by scholars in other fields, such as psychopathology and social, gender and cross-cultural psychology, who try to explain categorical differences in mentalization abilities. To illustrate, individuals with "autism spectrum disorder" are profoundly impaired in attributing mental states (Baron-Cohen et al., 1985). These impairments in mental state attribution were defined by Baron-Cohen (1990) as the "mindblindness theory" of autism.

There is evidence to believe that the development of mentalization, especially at higher levels, is closely linked to language development in humans. For instance, young children must possess an understanding of mental state words such as "think" and "believe" before they can make theory of mind inferences. Exposure to language helps children to become familiar with the various mental states and perspectives of others. There is also evidence that the neural networks responsible for language and those implicated in theory of mind reasoning are closely linked.

Mentalization depends not only on social processes and language, but also on our capacity for "cognitive control" and "cognitive flexibility." Many studies have found correlations between children's mentalization abilities and their performance on a variety of tests that measure executive functioning. "Executive functions" comprise a set of cognitive processes involved in attention, working memory, response inhibition, resistance to interference and planning. "Sharing of attention" with others is a hallmark of mentalization. In addition, executive functioning enables us to form "metarepresentations" of the content of our minds and those of others. Our ability to respond to others on the basis of their mental states (rather than our own) is *mediated* through executive functioning. Cognitive control and flexibility are particularly important in complex social situations that require the highest level of mentalization.

Additionally, "affect regulation" has been associated with our ability to mentalize, with research indicating that high levels of stress, boredom, or fight, flight and freeze states, significantly interfere with our capacity to mentalize during social interaction.

Moving away from scientific research to practical applications of mentalization, we see that in recent years psychotherapists have increasingly recognized mentalization as a fundamental component of psychotherapeutic treatments. In fact, mentalization is the *principal* and most *persistent* mental activity that a patient employs during psychotherapy. Patients mentalize when they narrate their reasons for seeking psychological help, when they explain how they experience situations, when they disclose details of their relationships with others, and so forth. Most importantly, patients *activate* and *develop* their ability to mentalize through the *associations* they make between their own behavior and the behavior of others, including their interactive behavior with the therapist. It is not only the patient, however, who mentalizes during therapy sessions; mentalization efforts are also employed by the therapist. Therapists are constantly trying to understand what is going on in their patients' minds, to gain insight into their mental states and behaviors and to find the most effective ways to change unhealthy patterns in their thought processes and behavior. Furthermore, therapists help patients to develop their mentalization abilities: first, to help them understand and navigate their own inner world; second, to help them understand and navigate the social world; and third, to better connect their inner world with the social world. A clinical therapy that focuses on mentalization in particular is known as "mentalization-based therapy" (MBT). The development of this therapy finds its roots in research on theory of mind in relation to children with autism spectrum disorders. More recently, therapeutic interventions of this nature have been extended to adult patient groups and to patient groups with other psychological disorders. "Adaptive mentalization-based integrative treatment" (AMBIT) is an extension of mentalization-based therapy. As with MBT, therapeutic interventions using AMBIT focus on patient groups with complex psychological problems, in particular people with "borderline personality disorder" (BPD). People who suffer from BPD comprise a population that represents extreme deficiencies in mentalization and affective communication. *Underdeveloped* mentalization abilities have serious implications in relation to the formation of attachment relationships and self-development, both problematic areas for people who suffer from BPD. Vice versa, the attachment relationships that we develop, especially with our primary caregivers during childhood, significantly influence the strength of our mentalization capacity. *Securely* attached individuals tend to have more complex and sophisticated mentalization abilities than *insecurely* attached individuals.

Both within and outside of the clinical field, another factor that presents unique challenges to our ability to mentalize about others is "sociocultural diversity." When we do not share the same values, customs, beliefs and social rules with someone else, mentalization becomes increasingly difficult, and the accuracy of our inferences decreases significantly. In particular, when two people do not speak the same language they have to rely heavily on nonverbal behavior, which itself is subject to cultural differences in encoding and decoding.

To conclude, mentalizing on a basic, affective and strategic level enables us to take, gain, shift and shape the perspectives of others and our own perspectives. Mentalization is integral to our capacity to understand others and to understand ourselves. It is the most *powerful social tool* that we have at our disposal, affecting our well-being on a social, psychological and physiological level. Vice versa, the ability to mentalize is affected by a wide array of *intra*personal, *inter*personal and *extra*personal factors, such as our motivation to mentalize, the person about whom we mentalize and the sociocultural environment in which we are mentalizing. Having well-developed mentalization abilities is associated with a multitude of social and personal advantages. However, before we can determine what our mentalization proficiency level is, we need to be able to recognize the indicators that evidence good or poor mentalizing. This is not only critical for estimating our own level of mastery, but also the level of those with whom we interact. Having well-developed mentalization skills yourself does not guarantee successful interactions with others, especially not with those who might be struggling with severely underdeveloped mentalization abilities. Besides recognizing good or poor mentalizing in others we need to be vigilant of those who use tactics that are indicative of "pseudomentalization." Mentalization is our most powerful social tool and its power invites certain people to use tricks that one easily mistakes for mentalization to manipulate us.

THE GOAL OF THIS BOOK

The goal of this book is twofold: first, *to introduce mentalization and theory of mind to the general public*, extending familiarity with these concepts, including the practice of mentalization, beyond the clinical and scientific environments; and second, *to provide a clear description of the theoretical foundation for mentalization*. In clinical settings, the focus lies primarily on developing mentalization to provide insight into both our inner world and the social environment, with the aim of making interpersonal interactions run more smoothly. There is, however, another level that is of great interest and equal value, namely the practical application of mentalization as a means of achieving strategic objectives.

In this book we provide you with guidance on applying mentalization efforts more effectively in your personal and professional dealings with others. We have translated the most current and influential scientific research on the subject matter into practical and applicable knowledge. Our extensive survey of literature on the subject of mentalization made us aware of the need to deconstruct this multifaceted ability into smaller conceptual pieces. This effort has yielded both a granular and a holistic explanation of what mentalization entails. Moreover, it has enabled us to develop multilayered mentalization assessment tools and offer services that are tailored to specific training needs. In sum, our hierarchical classification helps to identify strengths and weaknesses in our mentalization competencies and helps to explain where, when and how the different levels of mentalization are best applied.

This book is divided into five sections. In the first section, we provide you with a general understanding of what mentalization entails. In the second section, we cover basic mentalizing. This most primitive level of mentalization helps us, among other things, to connect with others - to build rapport and share experiences nonverbally - and to detect nonverbal signals and cues that have the power to influence mental states and consequent behavior. In the third section, we explore the intermediate level of mentalization, affective mentalizing, which allows us to regulate our affective states and to influence the affective states of others. It helps us to avoid fight, flight, or freeze reactions, enabling us to remain open minded and to take in all of the relevant social information for mental state reasoning. Affective mentalizing also helps us to repair and maintain healthy relationships through empathy, compassion and competent affective communication. In the fourth section, we examine the highest level of mentalization, strategic mentalizing. Strategic mentalizing is instrumental in enhancing affiliation and cooperation, in socially distancing from others, or in gaining competitive advantage. The fifth and final section, mastering mentalization, deals with the mastery of this powerful human capacity. Here we discuss opportunities for assessment and enhancement of mentalization competencies.

Each chapter of this book is divided into three parts: first, an introduction with a short anecdote or discussion of an illustrative topic to set the stage; second, an examination of the core principles of the chapter's subject matter; and third, a discussion of the advantages of, and possible impediments to, development or enhancement of the mentalization skills described in the chapter.

This book will introduce you to a number of concepts with which you may not be familiar. Therefore, we provide you with concise definitions of the relevant terms of art. Wherever possible, we use lexical definitions employed within the field of mentalization. Definitions employed in other related fields, or having varying connotations, are distinguished as appropriate. A clear understanding of the terminology is central to capturing the essence of mentalization. We hope you will find this book insightful and enjoyable to read. If you would like additional information on the subject matter, you can reach us through our website at www.appliedtom.com.

References

Baron-Cohen, S. (1990). Autism: A specific cognitive disorder of "mind-blindness." *International Review of Psychiatry, 2*, 79–88. https://doi.org/10.3109/09540269009028274

Baron-Cohen, S., Leslie, A. M., & Frith, U. (1985). Does the autistic child have a "theory of mind"? *Cognition, 21*, 37–46. doi:10.1016/0010-0277(85)90022-8

Dennett, D. C., (1971/1978) "Mechanism and Responsibility", reprinted in pp. 233–255 in Dennett, D. C., *Brainstorms: Philosophical Essays on Mind and Psychology*. Bradford Books 1978 (Montgomery) (originally published in 1971).

Dennett, D. C. (1987). *The Intentional Stance*. Cambridge, MA: MIT Press.

Descartes, R. (2008). *Meditations on first philosophy* (M. Moriarty, Trans.). Oxford University Press.

Frith, U., Morton, J., & Leslie, A. M. (1991). The cognitive basis of a biological disorder: autism. *Trends in Neurosciences, 14*(10), 433-438. doi:10.1016/0166-2236(91)90041-R

Goldman, A. I. (2006). *Simulating minds: The philosophy, psychology, and neuroscience of mindreading*. Oxford University Press. doi:10.1093/0195138929.001.0001

Gopnik, A., & Wellman, H. M. (1994). The theory theory. In L. A. Hirschfeld & S. A. Gelman (Eds.), *Mapping the mind: Domain specificity in cognition and culture* (pp. 257–293). Cambridge University Press. doi:10.1017/cbo9780511752902.011

Gordon, R. M. (1986). Folk Psychology as Simulation. *Mind and Language, 1*, 158–171.

Gordon, R. M. (1992). The Simulation Theory: Objections and Misconceptions. *Mind & Language, 7*(1-2), 11–34. doi:10.1111/j.1468-0017.1992.tb00195.x

Harris, P. L. (1992). From Simulation to Folk Psychology: The Case for Development. *Mind & Language, 7*(1-2), 120–144. doi:10.1111/j.1468-0017.1992.tb00201.x

Morton, A. (1980). *Frames of Mind*. Oxford University Press.

Premack, D., & Woodruff, G. (1978). Does the chimpanzee have a theory of mind? *Behavioral and Brain Sciences, 1*(4), 515–526. doi:10.1017/S0140525X00076512

Turing, A. M. (1950) Computing Machinery and Intelligence. *Mind, 49*, 433–460. doi:https://doi.org/10.1093/mind/LIX.236.433

Whiten, A. (Ed.). (1991). *Natural theories of mind: Evolution, development and simulation of everyday mindreading*. Basil Blackwell.

SECTION I.

MENTALIZATION

To Regard and Understand

Guilty or Not?

In the United States, the prosecution bears the burden of proving the guilt of a criminal defendant beyond a reasonable doubt. Thus, if the jury has reasonable doubt as to any material element of the crime, they are duty bound to find the defendant not guilty. A man has been charged with first degree murder, even though the police never found the victim's body. After a lengthy trial, the defense attorney concludes his closing argument by pointing to a clock on the wall and declaring: "*Ladies and gentlemen of the jury, in 10 seconds the alleged victim is going to walk right through that door.*" He then theatrically turns his attention toward the courtroom door. Everyone in the courtroom waits in suspense for the dramatic entry, but the victim never materializes. Feeling very pleased with himself, the defense attorney continues by saying: "*The very fact that you were all waiting for the victim to walk through that door establishes that there is reasonable doubt as to my client's guilt."* The jury retires to deliberate, only to return with a verdict in less than 30 minutes. The defense attorney is now more confident than ever that his clever ploy has worked to perfection. *"What is your verdict,"* the judge asks. *"Guilty,"* the jury foreman announces. The stunned defense attorney rises in protest and challenges the jury: *"But you were all looking at the door, waiting for the victim to appear! How could you possibly fail to have reasonable doubt?"* The jury foreman answers: *"Well, almost everybody in the courtroom may have been looking at the door, but I was looking at your client, and he definitely wasn't looking at the door, he was looking at us."*

What was it that made the jury foreman act differently than the rest of the jury members so that reasonable doubt evaporated? While it might have been tempting to follow the defense attorney's clever misdirection, the jury foreman realized that the key to solving the case was *understanding what was going on in the mind of the defendant.* He knew that if the defendant looked at the door, as the rest of the jury did, the defendant might himself have been expecting the victim to walk into the courtroom. The defendant, however, focused on the jury members to infer their mental states, hoping to determine if they had fallen for the courtroom theatrics of his defense attorney. By watching the defendant's reaction, the jury foreman concluded that the defendant did *not* expect the victim to walk through the door - knowing full well that the victim was dead. Instead, the defendant was looking at the jury members, hoping that they would find him not guilty, based on their own reasonable doubt.

This anecdote illustrates convincingly how the use of our mentalization abilities can provide us with the information we need to reach accurate conclusions about what is going on in the minds of others, a skill known as "interpersonal accuracy." "**Mentalization**" pertains to our ability to detect verbal and nonverbal signals and cues, and use them to infer mental states upon which we can base more fully-informed predictions and explanations of behavior. It entails taking the perspectives of others. "**Perspective taking**" involves noting physical changes in another person relative to their surroundings, taking their *vantage point*, while looking for affect and intent signals and cues in their nonverbal behavior. Mentalization also entails gaining the perspectives of others. "**Perspective gaining**" involves sharing the *conceptual viewpoint* of another person. We gain the perspectives of others through verbal or written information exchanges. Mentalization is critical to the ability to *shift* between different perspectives and to *compare* different mindsets to one another, which we refer to as "**perspective shifting**." Finally, mentalization is key to our ability to shape the perspectives of others. "**Perspective shaping**" entails the *conscious* and *controlled* use of mentalization to understand how to best impact the perspectives and accompanying behavior of other people in order to promote our objectives. The taking, gaining, shifting and shaping of the perspectives of others is known as "***inter*personal mentalizing**." Mentalization does not focus solely on the perspectives of others. We also mentalize about ourselves by taking our own perspectives, through the conscious observation of something of interest, and considering our affective, cognitive and behavioral response in relation to our observation. We gain our own perspectives by using our inner voice to reason about our own mental states. This "***intra*personal mentalizing**" is key to shifting our own perspectives, for example, comparing our own perspective to that of another, or moving from an old perspective to a new one. Intrapersonal mentalizing is also critical to shaping our own perspectives through internal monologues that help us arrive at a satisfying understanding of different situations. As with interpersonal mentalizing, we mentalize about our own mental states to explain and predict our own behavior. The ability to mentalize about ourselves is also referred to as "self-mentalizing."

Mental state reasoning extends even beyond intra- and interpersonal mentalizing. We use it to consider how extrapersonal factors, such as contextual and environmental influences, impact mental states in general. We refer to this aspect of mentalization as "***extra*personal mentalizing**." Additionally, extrapersonal mentalizing relates to reasoning about mental states on a group level. Here we mentalize about others with whom we do not have personal interaction. For instance, we consider predominantly shared mental states that may underlie the perspectives of people from different cultures. The process of taking, gaining, shifting and shaping perspectives of larger groups is similar to interpersonal mentalizing, although its scope is much broader.

We mentalize on the basis of signals and cues that we gather through the observation of others and ourselves. A "**signal**" is anything that intentionally changes or maintains the mental states and behavior of the recipient. A "**cue**" is anything that unintentionally changes or maintains the mental states and behavior of the recipient. Throughout this book we regularly use the word "indicators" to refer to both signals and cues. These "**social indicators**" can be obtained *directly* via observable behavior, for instance, a clear emotional expression or other nonverbal behavior. Alternatively, the information can be obtained *indirectly* via *non*-observable signals and cues that we extract from other sources, such as verbal accounts, and by the reactions that we detect in our own sensorial system in relation to those signals and cues. All of these indicators carry pieces of information that communicate meaning. Moreover, they have the capacity to influence the mental states and behavior of the recipient.

What is a mental state? A "**state of mind**" is the psychological state that a person has at a given time, or the condition or quality of a person's thoughts or feelings. We have classified mental states into four "**primary mental states**:" affect, desire, belief and knowledge. "**Affect**" pertains to our feelings, moods and emotions. Desire, belief and knowledge comprise our more "epistemic" - or cognitive - mental states. "**Desire**" is a strong feeling of wanting to have something (the affective side of desire), or a strong wish for something to happen (the cognitive side of desire). "**Belief**" refers to an acceptance that something exists or is true, especially without the need for proof. "**Knowledge**" pertains to facts, information and skills acquired through experience, education, or the theoretical or practical understanding of a subject. These four primary mental states influence one another significantly and therefore need to be considered in relation to one another.

For instance, desire and, to a lesser extent, beliefs are often closely linked to our affective mental states. Knowledge is the most purely cognitive of our mental states, and therefore the least impacted by our affect. The primary mental states can be viewed as the building blocks for secondary, "**complex mental states.**" Complex mental states include, for instance, "**intentions**" - having an aim or plan, "**attitudes**" - a settled way of thinking or feeling about something, and "**motivations**" - reasons for acting or behaving in a particular way, all of which guide our behavior. These complex mental states are thus composed of the four primary mental states. Mental states have the potential to convert thought into action. To illustrate, *I may feel frustrated* (affective state) *that I often don't understand other people well* (knowledge state by understanding lack of knowledge), *I want to change that* (desire state), *I believe that it is possible to do so* (belief state), and *I come to learn how I can read people better* (knowledge state). These four primary mental states together trigger and increase motivational and intentional considerations. And *now I am reading a book on mentalization* (action), which is the "behavioral consequence" of following up on those considerations. Complex mental states can be defined as the link between the primary mental states and the actual execution of behavior aimed at reaching a complex goal. Intentions, however, often are not acted upon (for all kinds of reasons), which presents a significant problem with regard to the predictability of behavior. Thus, before we can accurately predict what someone is going to do, we also need to account for factors that can influence a person's decision-making process. Competing mental states, other people and contextual and environmental factors, all exert strong and persistent influences on us, and those influences can have a decisive impact on whether or not our intentions and motivations will be acted upon.

These influential factors can be seen as moderators or mediators. "**Moderators**" are factors that *make the probability of behavior weaker or stronger*, for instance, the amount of energy someone has to act upon an intention. When we are tired, we are less likely to make the effort to gain accurate perspectives of others, but when we are well-rested we are more likely to devote the energy required to figure out what is truly going on in the minds of others. A "**mediator**" is a factor that *causes the behavior to either be carried out or not.* To illustrate, the salience, importance and ambiguity of a situation mediate the transition from casual interaction with others, to mentalizing about them. Therefore, when we are in an interview for our dream job, we will do our utmost to assess what the interviewer is looking for, in other words, we engage in "**concurrent mentalizing.**" In contrast, when we are in a cafe with a couple of friends after work discussing random topics, we do not perceive a need to bring our more effortful mentalization faculties online.

The mindful inferences, or theories, regarding intentions and motivations that we impute to others, including the consideration of mediators and moderators, constitute the bases upon which we predict future behavior. When we try to predict the future behavior of others - "**prospective mentalizing**" - we reason ahead based upon what we think is going on in their minds. This is called "**forward-chaining.**" For instance, the defense lawyer predicted that if he could change the collective mental state of the jury so that they believed the victim might walk into the courtroom, the jury might find the defendant not guilty on the basis of reasonable doubt. In predicting behavior, we move forward in time. This is called "**mental time travel**" - also known as "chronosthesia." Mental time travel is our capacity to mentally put ourselves in a past situation, to imagine an alternative scenario for the current situation, or to imagine a possible future scenario. Our mindful inferences, together with our ability for mental time travel, also help us to explain past behavior - "**retrospective mentalizing.**" When we are trying to explain past behavior, we move backward in our reasoning to consider the mental states that motivated behavior. This is known as "**backward-chaining.**" To illustrate, in criminal cases, investigators, attorneys, judges and juries apply backward-chaining to determine the factors upon which past behavior was based (their motive). In our interactions with others, we often reason both ways, forward and backward. Thus, this forward and backward chaining in mentalization is usually an *iterative* process. To be able to do this well we need to apply different competencies that work together to shape our mentalization proficiency.

Three Levels of Mentalization

Mentalization is a multi-faceted ability, which operates *simultaneously* and *dynamically* at multiple levels. For the sake of clarity, and to facilitate the assessment and training of mentalization skills, we have embraced a three-level hierarchical organization. We refer to the three constituent levels of mentalization as:

1. Basic mentalizing
2. Affective mentalizing
3. Strategic mentalizing

People navigate through these three levels of mentalization during their interactions with others. Our hierarchical classification helps to explain where, when and how the different levels of mentalization are best applied. It also helps to identify strengths and weaknesses in our mentalization competencies. We will now consider each level in detail. We start with the most elementary level: basic mentalizing.

BASIC MENTALIZING

Basic mentalizing encompasses the most elementary aspects of mentalization. It concerns our ability to detect social indicators as a result of changes we sense within ourselves due to our primitive tendency to share in affect and to synchronize our behavior with people around us through *mimicry, affective contagion* and *behavioral contagion.* This predisposition generally operates subconsciously, however, and we need to train ourselves to become aware of it as these primitive synchronizing abilities are critically important in understanding human cognition, affect and behavior in social interaction. Generally, we are more aware of the social signals and cues that we can detect in nonverbal behavior with our visual and auditory information processing channels. A part of our social information exchange, however, is revealed through our predisposition to mimic others and through changes in our interoceptive and exteroceptive sensorial system which operates predominantly on a subconscious level. Basic mentalizing further encompasses *the detection of nonverbal social indicators* – such as gestures, vocalics and facial expressions - *without the embodied sharing* found in mimicry, affective contagion and behavioral contagion. Finally, basic mentalizing includes *the sensing of nonsocial exteroceptive and interoceptive stimuli* – such as noise or fatigue - that do not transmit social information, but nevertheless have a considerable impact on our attentional focus and our interpretation of social indicators. Mentalizing on this level helps us:

- To infer people's basic affective mental states and straightforward elemental needs and intentions through their observable nonverbal behavior.
- To connect with others through nonverbal behavior, build rapport and create a positive ambiance so that they do not feel restrained in their nonverbal or verbal behavior.
- To facilitate smooth interaction and elicit prosocial behavior.
- To heighten the accuracy of our higher-level mentalization inferences.
- To stay aware of possible bias in our explanations and predictions of behavior through the monitoring of interoceptive and exteroceptive sensations.
- To be aware of our own inclination to "catch" the affective states of others, or to mimic their behavior.

There are several key aspects of basic mentalizing. Basic mentalizing is *embodied*; we feel it and act it out. Mentalizing on this level is often done *unconsciously* and *implicitly*. This level of mentalization is *always online*, meaning that it remains available throughout our interactions with others. Information sharing on this level is *nonverbal, intuitive* and *unplanned*. The advantages of mentalizing on this level are that it is *fast, effortless* and *continuous*. The disadvantages are that it is *primitive, limited* and *rigid*. The fact that basic mentalizing is an economical way of mentalizing comes with a tradeoff: it is *hard to control*, and the level of *accuracy* tends to be *low* in complex situations. We now continue to the second and intermediate level of mentalization, affective mentalizing.

AFFECTIVE MENTALIZING

Affective mentalizing refers to the level of mentalization at which we consciously monitor our own affective mental states, such as emotions, moods and feelings, and the affective mental states of others. This "conscious monitoring" allows us to regulate our own affective states and to influence those of others. Mentalizing at this level is critical to *defusing stressful and emotionally charged social interactions,* since mentalization in general is compromised by intense feelings. Stress and intense emotions tend to direct our attentional focus toward ourselves, preparing us for a fight, flight, or freeze reaction. Affective mentalizing is also critical to *assuring that our mentalization faculties do not lapse when we are too relaxed or fatigued.*

Affective mentalizing helps us to process the nonverbal affect signals and cues that we gather using our basic mentalizing skills. Additionally, it helps us to connect those *nonverbal* affect indicators to the *verbal* accounts by which people share their feelings, enhancing a mutual understanding of how a situation is experienced. On this level we apply our *empathic, compassionate* and *affective communication* competencies to regulate affective states, both our own and those of others. Affective mentalizing is, moreover, a prerequisite for strategic mentalizing, in which this affective information is incorporated into increasingly rational models of people's intentions and motivations.

There are several important aspects of affective mentalizing. Simulation and projection are two key features of our mentalization efforts on the affective level. "**Simulation**" involves sharing in the affect of others in order to better understand how they experience a situation. "**Projection**," on the other hand, involves a cognitive effort to understand the affective mental states of others by "projecting" ourselves into the same situation, while using *our own* feelings, thoughts and experiences as a proxy for those of others. This projection is the core idea of what is meant by "*putting yourself in the shoes of another person.*" Simulation is initiated below our level of consciousness through mimicry, affective contagion and behavioral contagion, and is subsequently applied to empathize with others. Projection, on the other hand, requires conscious thought from the outset. Both simulation and projection are essential prerequisites for empathizing with others. Through simulation and projection, we can be very effective in understanding and dealing with emotions. Affective mentalizing does *not* require consideration and evaluation of increasingly rational models in order to be effective, as is the case with strategic mentalizing.

Although we specifically mention simulation and projection as key features of affective mentalizing, this does not mean that affective mentalizing encompasses only these two features. Many of the key features of basic and strategic mentalizing are represented in this intermediate level as well, although to a more moderate degree, and with a particular focus on affective mental states. Affective mentalizing is, for instance, *slower than basic mentalizing and more effortful*. On the other hand, *it is faster than strategic mentalizing,* though in complex circumstances, *more prone to error*. The primary focus of affective mentalizing is restoring affective states. Once affective states are restored to a well-balanced level, we can redirect our focus from relational goals to more instrumental goals.

STRATEGIC MENTALIZING

Strategic mentalizing is the highest and most cognitive level of mentalization where we form a theory of mind about what is going on in the minds of others. "**Theory of mind**" is a term used in scientific research to refer to the capacity to mentalize about other people's increasingly epistemic (cognitive) mental states, such as desires, beliefs and knowledge, and complex mental states such as intentions, motivations and attitudes. This level of mentalization enables us to *look beyond observable informational signals and cues to develop increasingly rational theories of what is going on in the minds of others.* We refer to this level as "strategic mentalizing" since *it involves the prediction or explanation of increasingly complex goal-directed behavior*. It generally implicates mentalizing to *infer the intention or motivation of people to either affiliate and cooperate, or to socially distance and compete.*

The concept of strategic mentalizing can be distinguished from basic and affective mentalizing in terms of "**metacognitive processes**," processes that entail thinking about how people think. Aspects of strategic mentalizing overlap to a certain extent with metacognitive thinking, as theory of mind reasoning is a *form* of metacognitive thinking. It is at this intersection of cognitive analysis where we advance from common-sense inferences to more critical reasoning that is grounded in psychological and sociological theoretical models and empirical research findings. Strategic mentalizing provides us with the capacity to test our common-sense inferences against alternative models of, or explanations for, human behavior. In contrast to basic mentalizing, which focuses on nonverbal behavior to take the perspectives of others, and affective mentalizing, which primarily concerns the reflection of affective mental states by simulation or projection, strategic mentalizing focuses on the epistemic mental states largely obtained through *verbal* information sharing. In other words, strategic mentalizing enables us to *gain* the "cognitive" perspectives of others. It is on this strategic level that verbal communication becomes a strong focal point, since the more cognitive mental states cannot be inferred through observation alone. Nonetheless, basic mentalizing and affective mentalizing still play a pivotal role in our understanding of the minds of others, and therefore factor into strategic mentalizing as well. Affect indicators are, for instance, processed during affective *theory of mind* reasoning where we use this affective information to predict or explain behavior.

What are the key features of our mentalization efforts on this highest level? Strategic mentalizing is *cognitive, conscious,* and *explicit.* This level of mentalization is generally *offline,* and must be either triggered by external events, or consciously brought online. It is often employed outside of the immediate interaction, either to prepare for social encounters beforehand, or to evaluate them after the fact. The information flow is *verbal, rational, strategic* and *specific to the individual.* The advantages of mentalizing on this level are that it is *complex, sophisticated* and *flexible,* which significantly enhances accuracy in complex situations. Furthermore, we have a *high level of control* over this mentalization level. The limitations of strategic mentalizing are that it is *slow, deliberative* and *more effortful*.

One final remark on strategic mentalizing is that theory of mind reasoning is *not* synonymous with "social intelligence." Although forming alliances and behaving strategically with others can be viewed as evidence of social intelligence, it is not necessarily evidence of an understanding of what is going on in the minds of others. For theory of mind, we need evidence of mental state inferences and behavior tailored to that understanding. To illustrate, when a teacher recognizes that a student does not grasp a concept, the teacher needs to consider what approaches might work better for this particular person's learning style, and tailor his or her teaching methodology accordingly. Nevertheless, mentalization does bolster our social intelligence significantly, and vice versa.

Six Dimensions of Mentalization

Now that we have examined mentalization on three different levels, it should be apparent that mentalization is not only a multi*level* ability, it is also a multi*dimensional* ability. Six dimensions of mentalization can be distinguished, four of which are based upon findings by Lieberman (2007), and further applied in the field of clinical psychology by Bateman and Fonagy (2016) in their book *Mentalization-Based Treatment for Personality Disorders*. In our research, we have identified two additional dimensions that are relevant to mentalization. As Bateman and Fonagy mention, mentalization dimensions are useful in creating a personal mentalization profile. They can be viewed as spectra that can be used to assess mentalization competencies in terms of our position on a scale ranging between two extremes. Each individual pole on a given spectrum is important for comprehensive mentalizing, however, we need to apply the right specific directional focus and level of effort at the right time and within the right context. We will now continue with an explanation of each dimension in relation to our three-level model of mentalization, starting with four dimensions that are based on those identified by Lieberman, Bateman and Fonagy.

The first dimension, "**cognitivity**," pertains to the spectrum ranging from "*intuitive*" to "*reasoned*" mentalizing. At the elementary level, basic mentalizing, our impressions are largely spontaneous, and we apply intuitive processes to infer the mental states of others. At the highest level, strategic mentalizing, we use reasoned, critical thinking processes to infer the mental states of others. When it comes to affective mentalizing, we operate more or less in the middle of the spectrum, utilizing both verbal and nonverbal social indicators, primarily to infer affective mental states through simulation or projection. Both intuitive and reasoned mentalizing are important and beneficial, provided we apply them at the right time and within the right context.

The second dimension, "**indicator focus**," ranges from "*observed external*" to "*inferred internal*" mentalizing. This dimension refers to our tendency to infer mental states in a given situation based upon external indicators that we detect in the behavior of others (or in our own behavior when we self-mentalize) versus our tendency to infer mental states on the basis of what we know about the other person (or ourselves). Here, the distinction between basic and strategic mentalizing is once again reflected. Whereas with basic mentalizing we focus on nonverbal signals and cues conveyed by a person together with the contextual indicators that we can see, hear, feel and even smell, with strategic mentalizing we look for clues in self-disclosure and narratives to infer nonobservable elements. Once again, affective mentalizing lies between those two extremes on the spectrum with the focus limited to affective mental states.

The third dimension, "**mental state focus**," encompasses the continuum from "*affective focused*" to "*cognitive focused*" mentalizing. This dimension refers to our tendency to make mental state inferences on the basis of social indicators that signal emotions, feelings and moods, versus mental state inferences based on social indicators that signal such cognitive mental states as intention, knowledge, or belief. Affective focused mentalizing, as the term suggests, relates primarily to the affective mentalizing level. Cognitive focus, on the other hand, involves the ability to reason about the more cognitive mental states of belief, desire and knowledge in order to explain and predict behavior, and relates primarily to the strategic mentalizing level. Some people, for instance, explain experiences purely from a rational point of view ignoring any reference to affective experiences.

The fourth dimension, "**person focus**," ranges from "*self-focused*" to "*other-focused*" mentalizing. During the process of mentalization we need to focus on ourselves and our objectives, while at the same time remaining mindful of others and their objectives, an ability we refer to as "perspective shifting."

We have added a fifth dimension, "**effort balance**," as it is instructive to examine mentalization extremes ranging from "*hypermentalizing*" to "*hypomentalizing*." When we mentalize constantly at maximum capacity, or when we neglect to mentalize when it is called for, our interactions with others will leave us with unsatisfying results, or even worse, render us socially isolated. Both extremes, hyper- and hypomentalizing, can be suggestive of a psychological disorder or a physiological impairment. Here again, achieving the right balance is key to effective mentalizing.

Finally, we have added a sixth dimension, "**mentalizing orientation**," which refers to the detection of our dialectical behavioral tendencies either to show prosocial intent and behavior to affiliate and cooperate with others, or to demonstrate antisocial intent and behavior to socially distance from, or compete against, others. Thus, this spectrum ranges from "*affiliate/cooperate*" to "*socially distance/compete*." Strategic mentalizing focuses on these two basic modes of social interaction. While affiliation/cooperation refers to the action or process of associating with others and working together to the same end, social distancing/competition pertains to the action or process of dissociating from others and striving to gain or win something, or prevailing over others. This level of mentalization requires monitoring of not only one's own actions, but also the actions of others, as well as adopting a specific mental set, as Decety et al. (2004) describe in their research on neural bases of cooperation and competition. This assertion was corroborated by these scholars with their identification of "distinct [brain] regions to be selectively associated with cooperation and competition whereby neurological patterns reflect the different mental frameworks implicated in being cooperative versus competitive with another person." Let us explore the neurological underpinnings of mentalization a bit more.

Neurological Underpinnings of Mentalization

Not all of the cognitive processes associated with mentalization evolved at the same time. Mentalization components were built upon preexisting neural systems for primitive social interaction. However, not all neural systems required for mentalization came into being for social interaction. For instance, "executive functions" - our neural systems for attention, working memory and goal directedness - are needed to facilitate mentalization, but they serve *non*social objectives as well. For example, our working memory is crucial for solving puzzles, but it is also essential for perspective shifting, which involves mentalizing about others while keeping our own perspective in mind. When we examine the evolutionary history of the development of mentalization, we see that the ability to detect nonverbal mental state indicators developed before our ability to detect verbal mental state indicators. In addition, we find the same developmental sequence in the way children develop their mentalization competencies, a phenomenon that we will address later in this chapter. This developmental sequence is also reflected in the three levels of mentalization as illustrated below.

We can visualize the different levels of mentalization - basic, affective and strategic - in terms of a distributed brain network supporting mentalization. From an evolutionary point of view, primal brain regions involved in basic mentalizing emerged earlier than the core brain structures for affective processing implicated in our neurological network for affective mentalizing. Strategic mentalizing depends more on neurological networks that involve our most recently developed cerebral architecture. We need to keep in mind, however, that brain structures are heavily interlinked in functional networks, and it is not possible to discuss the brain regions that we associate with different mentalization levels in isolated terms. Moreover, brain regions that are involved in mentalization are not necessarily exclusively devoted to reading minds. Finally, several brain regions are merely supportive of mentalization, as they are part of a domain-general network rather than a domain-specific one.

NEUROLOGICAL UNDERPINNINGS OF BASIC MENTALIZING

As basic mentalizing is our most elementary mentalization level, it involves the more primal structures of our brain, such as:

- The "**brainstem**," an area at the base of the brain structurally continuous with the cervical spinal cord. This brain structure serves a critical role in regulating attention, awareness and certain involuntary actions of the body, including heartbeat and breathing (Basinger & Hogg, 2020). The brain stem is part of the basal areas that are involved in recreating in one person the physiological state of another through affective mimicry and affective contagion.
- The "**basal ganglia**," a group of subcortical nuclei linked to the thalamus in the base of the brain, is involved in motor control and motor learning, executive functions, emotions and motivation. Additionally, it is involved in attentional allocation and filtering, acting as a selective gateway for the information that finds its way into working memory (Ring, 2002). Working memory content, particularly social information, is critical for perspective taking, gaining and shifting.
- The "**cerebellum**," a part of the brain at the back of the skull, coordinates and regulates muscular activity. Cerebellum structures control our innate and automatic self-preservation behavior pattern,

ensuring our survival. Other notable behavior patterns controlled by the cerebellum include nonverbal communication, and *socially-approved* motor activity, such as handshakes, head nods and bowing. Interestingly, recent research by Van Overwalle et al. (2014) found that "the cerebellum is implicated in social processes of 'body' reading (mirroring, e.g., understanding other persons' intentions from observing their movements) and 'mind' reading (mentalizing, e.g., inferring other persons' beliefs, intentions or personality traits, reconstructing persons' past, future, or hypothetical events)." These researches added that "[t]hese cerebellar functions are connected with corresponding functional networks in the cerebrum.

- The "**anterior insula**," at the front of the insular cortex is a portion of the cerebrum involved in consciousness and diverse functions generally linked to affects, visceral information processing, interoception and the regulation of the body's homeostasis, empathy, perception, self-awareness and interpersonal experience. Uddin et al. (2017) explain the importance of the insula in socioemotional processing, particularly for interoceptive awareness to subjective emotional experiences. With regard to empathy and social cognition, these researchers write that "studies enlighten the important role of the left anterior insula in social affect, such as empathy, to distinguish primordial emotions like disgust, fear, and happiness."
- The "**anterior cingulate cortex**," the frontal part of the cingulate cortex (a part of the brain situated in the medial aspect of the cerebrum), is implicated in the detection and appraisal of social processes, including social exclusion, conflict monitoring and error detection. Apps et al. (2016) found that this brain structure "plays a crucial role in evaluating the behaviors of others and in estimating others' level of motivation." Additionally, the anterior cingulate cortex plays an important role in registering and monitoring not only physical pain, but also, as proposed by Eisenberger (2003), *social* or *emotional* pain. For instance, the social distancing efforts of a

person can trigger this sort of "psychological" pain in the person or group at whom such efforts are directed.

- "**Mirror neurons**" are linked to action recognition, understanding of manual gestures, understanding the goal of an action (intention) and imitating behavior (including mimicry and behavioral contagion) (see Keysers & Gazzola, 2006; Rizzolatti & Sinigaglia, 2008). Brain regions commonly involved in imitation are the superior parietal lobule, inferior parietal lobule and the dorsal part of the premotor cortex (Molenberghs et al., 2009). Nonverbal behaviors and their accompanying sounds inform us about mental states. Because mirror neurons are recruited when we merely think about actions, they will likely show increased activity when we try to predict or explain another's behavior, and therefore they are involved in higher-level mentalizing as well. In relation to affective mimicry and its frequently concomitant, affective contagion, Bastiaansen et al. (2009) suggest that "[m]otor simulation may be a trigger for the simulation of associated feeling states." These researchers posit that the simulation of affective states involves "a mosaic of affective, motor and somatosensory components."

NEUROLOGICAL UNDERPINNINGS OF AFFECTIVE MENTALIZING

With regard to affective mentalizing, it is important to focus on the involvement of the limbic system, which, together with multiple lower and higher order systems, is heavily implicated in processing feelings, moods and emotions, as well as the affective aspects of desires and other more cognitive mental states. The "**limbic system**" is a collection of brain structures located in the middle of the brain that are concerned with affect and instinct. This system is involved in the processing of basic emotions (e.g., sadness, anger, happiness) and drives (e.g., hunger, thirst, sex, care of offspring). The brain structures in the limbic system are also involved in motivation, memory and learning, providing the capacity for greater flexibility in our behavior. In addition, the limbic system plays a crucial role in the formation of affective attachment relationships with others (Laurita et al. 2019). A few examples of the constituent brain structures of the limbic system are:

- The "**amygdala**," a roughly almond-shaped mass of grey matter inside each cerebral hemisphere, that is involved, among other things, in the detection and recognition of emotional facial expressions, vocal tones and body postures, and in the processing of social information more generally (Eslinger et al., 2001). The amygdala is one part of the brain mechanism that underlies empathy and allows for "affective attunement." It also creates the pathway for mimicry and affective contagion.
- The "**thalamus**," the superior part of the brainstem lying between the cerebral hemispheres on either side of the third ventricle, relays sensory information and acts as a center for pain perception. The thalamus is related to the perception, experience and recollection of affective states. It is also activated when predicting affective states in others (Hooker et al., 2008).
- The "**hippocampus**," located in the inner (medial) region of the temporal lobe, is thought to be especially critical for learning, memory and spatial navigation. It is increasingly emerging as a part of the "moral brain." Rubin et al. propose in their 2014 article that the "hippocampus also plays a critical role by forming and reconstructing relational memory representations that underlie flexible cognition and social behavior."

NEUROLOGICAL UNDERPINNINGS OF STRATEGIC MENTALIZING

In relation to strategic mentalizing, there are several neural regions, all of them implicated in high-level cognitive functions, that are indicated as belonging to a "theory of mind network." In literature authored by Apperly (2011), and Baron-Cohen et al. (2013), the following key brain systems for theory of mind reasoning have been described:

- The "**medial prefrontal cortex**," a midline region in the prefrontal cortex, that in relation to mentalization is associated with self-processing (self-reflection) and other-processing, episodic memory, forming scripts of social events and emotional memory schemas (Van Overwalle, 2009).

- The "**temporo-parietal junction**" (TPJ), a bilateral brain region located at the intersection of the superior temporal sulcus, the inferior parietal lobe and the lateral occipital cortex, that is crucial for several aspects of "social cognition." It is, for instance, critical for *self-other distinction* processes and in processing *different perspectives,* both mental and spatial. To illustrate, the TPJ is activated when people consider the strategies of other players in a game. While the right TPJ is specifically associated with thinking about mental state content (i.e., a particular desire or belief), the left TPJ is associated with thinking about perspectives (e.g., Speitel et al., 2019; Geng & Vossel, 2013).
- The "**precuneus,**" a medial aspect of the posterior parietal lobe, that is involved in a variety of complex functions including episodic memory retrieval, self-related mental representations, first-person perspective taking (intrapersonal mentalizing), cue reactivity, the integration of information relating to perception of the environment, visual imagery and affective responses to pain (e.g., Fletcher et al., 1995; Lundstrom et al., 2005; Cavanna & Trimble, 2006).
- The "**posterior cingulate cortex,**" which is part of the default mode network (see below), is a functionally heterogeneous cortex important for the integration of information drawn from memory and/or perception including the perceptions of social dynamics (Leech et al., 2012; Leech & Sharp, 2014). It is involved in regulating the balance between internally and externally-focused attention, making it a crucial structure in awareness and attentional focus (Leech & Sharp, 2014). It plays a central role in supporting internally-directed cognition and is recruited for future thinking, mentalization and the recall of memories that have an emotional quality such as autobiographical memories (e.g., Brewer & Whitfield-Gabrieli, 2013;

Spreng et al., 2009). Additionally, it is associated with both meditation and mind wandering (Brewer & Garrison, 2014).

- The "**superior temporal sulcus**," which lies above the superior temporal gyrus, is crucial for numerous aspects of mentalization, such as biological motion perception, language understanding, processing of faces, reflecting on the mental states of others, cognitive empathy and perspective-taking (Hein & Knight, 2008).
- The "**temporal poles**," an association cortex situated at the anterior end of the temporal lobes, is involved in processing interoceptive sensory stimuli (bodily states such as hunger and fatigue), and intentional and emotional mental states and social concepts (a type of semantic memory). The left temporal pole is associated with language functions, including semantic processing (i.e., remembering names correctly) and speech comprehension, and the right temporal pole is related to personal and episodic memories. It is more closely associated with emotion and socially relevant memory, and it is involved in evaluating the emotional importance of sensory stimuli (see Herlin et al., 2021).

The brain regions associated with theory of mind reasoning find considerable overlap with the "**default mode network**" (DMN). Smallwood et al. (2021) describe the DMN as "a set of widely distributed brain regions in the parietal, temporal and frontal cortex," that "shows reductions in activity during attention-demanding tasks but increase their activity across multiple forms of complex cognition, many of which are linked to memory or abstract thought." The DMN is activated when our brain is in the so-called "resting" state. This happens when we focus on our internal mental-state processes (self-reflection, interoception, contemplating the future, meditation), or when we reason about the mental states of others, as opposed to focusing on the external world or on attention-demanding tasks (e.g., Spreng et al., 2009; Spreng & Grady, 2010; Brewer et al., 2011). This makes sense considering the fact that, particularly on the level of strategic mentalizing, we need to turn our intention inward to consider all the information at our disposal and rotate different perspectives in our working memory in order to accurately predict and explain behavior and to consciously adjust our behavior based on the inferences that we draw. At the lowest level of mentalization, basic mentalizing, our attention is largely directed to our external environment for purposes of detecting and collecting relevant social information.

We have to keep in mind that identifying brain regions and neurological networks that are linked to mentalization, or any other cognitive ability for that matter, is not straightforward or easy. Each mentalization level recruits brain regions that overlap with other mentalizing levels. As science continues to unravel the neurological underpinnings for mentalization, there will be adjustments and refinement of our understanding.

Development of Mentalization

Mentalization competencies are thus dependent upon the development of various brain structures and the functionality that those structures provide. The structures and functionality for basic mentalizing begin to develop in utero. Interestingly, research indicates that during pregnancy a mother's moods affect the unborn child's affective states, which in turn impact its neurobehavioral development (Kinsella & Monk, 2009), influencing the outcome of the child's mentalization abilities. There are different schools of thought with regard to the origins of behavioral contagion. On the one hand, there are studies supporting the proposition that imitation is innate (Meltzoff & Decety, 2003), while other research suggests that imitation is not an innate behavior, but rather one that is learned in a child's first months of life, even going so far as to propose that infants might learn to mimic the behavior of others by watching others mimic them (Oostenbroek et al., 2016). Regardless of whether imitation is innate or learned, soon after birth basic mentalizing takes off from the moment an infant can distinguish between self and others, enabling the infant to understand that it is imitating another person. Moreover, in order to engage in basic mentalizing, the infant needs to grasp the concept that the behaviors of others are *meaningful*, i.e., that the behaviors symbolize something.

Affective mentalizing emerges once children are able to appreciate affects and the affective aspect of desires. This is already observed at the age of two or three. We can infer affective mentalizing from the prosocial behavior that children display known as "targeted helping," defined by De Waal (2008) as "help and care based on a cognitive appreciation of the other's specific need or situation."

The development of strategic mentalizing begins with theory of mind reasoning skills that children acquire between the ages of four and five. It is during this developmental period that children start to understand the more cognitive mental states of desire, belief and knowledge. Researchers on theory of mind development in children divide mentalization abilities into implicit and explicit theory of mind reasoning. "Implicit theory of mind reasoning" pertains to behavioral predictions, whereby the child takes the mental state of others into account without deliberately reflecting on it. This is indicated as the "socio-perceptual" component of mentalization, which is an elementary form of mentalization, and therefore closely related to basic mentalizing. "Explicit theory of mind reasoning" is referred to as a deliberate consideration (e.g., a judgment) of mental states when predicting behavior. This is the "socio-cognitive" component of mentalization, an advanced form of mentalization and therefore closely related to strategic mentalizing. These concepts of theory of mind reasoning are, however, different from our definition of strategic mentalizing, as for young children, theory of mind reasoning is still a more basic endeavor. Both implicit and explicit theory of mind reasoning at this level of development does not yet involve the formation of increasingly rational models of what is going on in the minds of others based on complex psychological and sociological insights, as people are capable of doing when they get older. At this relatively early developmental stage, mentalization is still more akin to a form of "common-sense" psychology. Only after mentalizing becomes increasingly rational and strategic, enabling deliberations that move beyond the confines of rudimentary common-sense reasoning, is it possible to make mental state inferences and behavioral predictions based on the full-fledged theory of mind reasoning necessary for strategic mentalizing. Let us take a closer look at the sequence of theory of mind development in children as proposed by studies on the subject.

As with other cognitive skills, theory of mind competencies develop in a predictable, sequential pattern in normal child development. These sequences have been identified by using the "theory of mind scale," known as the ToM scale, developed by Wellman and Liu (2004) . The developmental sequence for theory of mind inferences starts when children are around three years old. The sequence is fully developed when the child is about seven years old. Generally speaking, the sequence progresses as follows:

- First, the child starts to understand that people can have "different desires" for the same thing.
- Later, the child understands that people can hold "different beliefs" about the same situation.
- Still later, the child grasps the idea that people can know something, but that others do not necessarily have the same knowledge (a concept known as "knowledge access").
- Next, the child develops an understanding of "false beliefs," knowing that something is true, but understanding that other people may falsely believe something different.
- And finally, the child develops the understanding that someone can feel a certain way, but display a "different emotional expression."

Interestingly, the general sequence of development for theory of mind competency in children is influenced in part by cultural background. For instance, researchers discovered that in China and Iran preschoolers first develop the understanding of knowledge access and later the understanding that people can hold different beliefs (Wellman et al., 2011; Shahaeian et al., 2014).

Contributing Mental Functions

There are two foundational abilities that are essential for mentalization. The first one is "**cognitive self-regulation**," which results from well-developed executive functions. The term "executive functions" pertains to a set of cognitive processes that are necessary for "cognitive control" (maintaining sustained attention, keeping working memory online, exercising impulse control, goal-directedness, etc.) and "cognitive flexibility" (changing attentional focal points, rotating alternative perspectives in working memory, etc.). The higher-order executive functions, involving multiple basic executive functions, are used for reasoning, problem solving and metacognitive thinking, and therefore are pivotal for strategic mentalizing. Cognitive self-regulation, in sum, concerns the process and components involved in deciding what to think, say and do. Cognitive self-regulation encompasses "affect regulation." This pertains to our ability to balance our affective sensations and to respond effectively to a situation by choosing the best affective response from the available alternatives. These responses should be sufficiently flexible to allow for spontaneous reaction, or for the selection of more appropriate reactions, taking the context into account.

The second ability is "**language**." Mentalization, in particular mentalizing at the strategic level, also depends on our capacity for language. Scholars postulate that the interface between language and mentalization is *bidirectional*. Both language and mentalization are complex and multifaceted systems. Moreover, the different components of each system can have varying relationships with components of the other systems. To make things even more complicated, these relationships can change over the course of a person's development. There is strong evidence to believe that both mentalization and language *depend on each other* to achieve their developmental potential, as studies with deaf children have indicated. When a deaf child is raised by parents who can hear, the child's mentalization capacity is often *under*developed as the communication between the child and its parents is limited, although this can be improved through training. When a deaf child is raised by at least one parent who also has a hearing impairment, the deaf child's mentalization ability is generally developed to a level equivalent to that of non-hearing impaired children, as both parent and child are similarly well versed in sign language, and therefore their communication is not limited. It is important to distinguish language in general from "mentalistic" language, which predominantly uses terms that refer to mental states such as beliefs, desires and intentions. The ability to use mentalistic language depends upon a good understanding of the *social meaning* of words that refer to mental states and the mind. We need to be able to have conversations with others about what they are *thinking* and *feeling*, and about what is going on in our own minds, as most, if not all, of this information is not directly inferable through nonverbal behavior. Conversely, our ability to use language effectively to influence our social environment is heavily dependent upon our understanding of how the minds of others work.

Thus, we understand from current research that mentalization is a *naturally developing system*, in that it develops naturally as our brain structures mature. To some degree, however, it is also a *developmental achievement* influenced by environmental factors such as:

- Caregiver's parenting style
- Presence or absence of siblings
- Experiences with peers
- Exposure to storybooks, cartoons and movies

Additionally, we need to view mentalization not only as a *trait* but also as a *state*. It is a trait in the sense that it relates to an individual's brain and personality development. It is also a state in that it is impacted by contextual aspects such as stress and arousal, the nature of relationships with others and other situational contingencies.

Mentalization Competencies: Advantages, Impediments and Avenues for Enhancement

Now that we have provided a general overview of the fundamental aspects of mentalization, we continue with a summary of the key advantages of possessing well-developed mentalization competencies, followed by a discussion of the impediments to developing these abilities. These advantages and impediments can impact people on three levels: *intra*personal, *inter*personal and *extra*personal. We will use these three categories throughout the book, as they represent the range of dimensional experiences across which mentalization skills can be applied. At the "***intra*****personal**" level, we focus on how mentalization affects us personally. At this level we also examine how our psychophysiological makeup affects our ability to mentalize. We examine intrapersonal factors to find out, for instance, how mentalization affects our sense of agency and self-efficacy, and how our temperament can promote or impede our mentalization practices. At the "***inter*****personal**" level, we examine how mentalization fosters good communication and healthy relationships. Additionally, we consider the interpersonal dynamics that either promote or impede our ability to mentalize. Thus, at the interpersonal level, the focus is on interactions between people, for example, negotiations, job interviews, the formation of new relationships, etc. At the "***extra*****personal**" level, we explore how mentalization brings about a better understanding of the world around us, beyond our interpersonal interactions. Moreover, we consider how extrapersonal factors (contextual and environmental effects) influence our mentalization ability. These factors have the capacity to moderate our mentalization efforts (making them stronger or weaker). They can also mediate our mentalization efforts, causing them to come online or be taken offline altogether. To illustrate, when you are interested in someone, your motivation to mentalize about that person increases, whereas a noisy environment or time pressure can disrupt mentalization activities. Let us take a look at the key advantages of well-developed mentalization skills on each level.

ADVANTAGES

Intrapersonally, *self-focused mentalizing helps us to understand ourselves better.* Studies show that people who are good at intrapersonal mentalizing tend to have excellent psychological and physiological awareness and understanding, sharpened goal directedness and a strong sense of "self-efficacy" (the belief in our innate ability to solve a problem, reach a goal, complete a task, or achieve what we set out to do). Mentalization can be seen as a feedback loop. In other words, from our interactions with others we learn how people think, feel and behave, and the way they react to us teaches us a great deal about our own thoughts, feelings and behaviors. A good self-understanding is critical to connecting and interacting effectively with others, which in turn strengthen our sense of "agency" - the capacity to act independently, make our own free choices, and exert control over situations.

On an interpersonal level, *mentalization competencies promote our understanding of others, including their subconscious, emotional and rational decision-making behavior.* This understanding is essential for predicting and explaining behavior. Moreover, a better understanding of others yields more fulfilling interactions and relationships. People appreciate us more when we understand them, and we are better able to affiliate with others and engage in cooperative behavior. Additionally, gaining a better understanding of others can provide us with a competitive advantage, and it helps us decide whether we would be wise to socially distance ourselves from others who do not have our best interests in mind.

Extrapersonally, we see that *people with well-developed mentalization competencies are also better at understanding people in general.* They are, for instance, the first to recognize a new trend, or to predict the long-term consequences of a leadership style on an organization. Accomplished mentalizers take contextual and environmental variables (e.g., a noisy environment, the influence of a large crowd, intercultural rules and regulations, etc.) into account in assessing their impact on interactions.

Mentalization is the most powerful social tool we have for navigating the social waters. We do, however, have to be mindful of potential impediments to mentalization. For instance, according to Hatfield et al. (1994), "People naturally attend consciously to only a small part of information being processed from moment to moment." Moreover, the stimuli that we do detect often are *not* the most indicative of the mental states of others. Let us look at the impediments to mentalization.

IMPEDIMENTS

Intrapersonally, *an individual's "genetic predisposition" can impede mentalizing willingness and accuracy*. For instance, a nervous temperament can interfere with accurate detection and interpretation of signals and cues. *Personality traits, which emerge from the confluence of temperament and social experiences, can arrest the development of mentalization competencies. Mental states that precede, or arise during, social interaction can likewise create mentalization challenges.* For instance, when another person becomes highly emotional, we may find it hard to keep from getting into the same emotional turmoil, with the result that our mentalization faculties are disrupted or taken offline altogether. Both *over*stimulation and *under*stimulation can *decrease* our capacity to mentalize about others. These factors turn our attention toward ourselves or away from social interaction. *Physical and psychological challenges may also contribute to mentalization difficulties.* When one of our senses is compromised (for example, if we cannot hear well), our ability to mentalize is significantly impaired. All of these challenges can impede mentalization, and our impaired mentalizing can, in turn, aggravate these challenges. Mentalization deficiencies have been identified as contributing to a range of mental and developmental disorders such as schizophrenia and autism. Personality disorders can have a significant impact on mentalization capacity. To illustrate, a person with social anxiety or borderline personality disorder tends to be too vigilant in their mentalization efforts, and often makes inaccurate inferences as to what is going on in the minds of others. People with antisocial personality traits often are able to mentalize strategically about others, but they lack, or fail to use, empathic feelings to guide their behavior in a prosocial manner. Alternatively, these people might use their empathic understanding with nefarious intent. Finally, we may sometimes have a hard time "switching off" our mentalization efforts, even when the context does not call for mentalizing. Many social interactions are automatic, such as paying for groceries at the checkout counter, and there isn't anything to be gained from analyzing the mental state of the cashier. While this is not an impediment or limitation to mentalization, it does deplete our available cognitive resources, and this "overthinking" can cause us to desynchronize with people around us, resulting in clumsiness or awkward social behavior.

Interpersonal impediments can exist within the context of social interaction as well. *The people with whom we interact play a crucial role in our mentalizing motivation.* For instance, when our relationship with a person is strained, or when we have no interest in talking to them, we are less inclined to mentalize about them to any significant degree. Differences in personal aspects such as status, cultural background, or age can also impact our level and degree mentalization. For instance, people of a *lower* social status tend to mentalize *more* about people of a higher status than vice versa. Gaining the perspective of a person with a different cultural or socioeconomic background can be very challenging. These differences can significantly increase the chances for verbal and nonverbal miscommunication and misunderstanding. Sometimes we can get too focused on our instrumental goals and forget about relational goals that allow us to remain on good terms with others.

On an extrapersonal level, one significant impediment to mentalization can be *physical distance.* Personal interaction via social media, email and communication applications such as Zoom or Skype can deprive us of opportunities to gather all of the data that we need for effective mentalizing. Another possible impediment is *situational context.* For instance, during a job interview, the interviewee has a limited opportunity to gather information about the interviewer, and therefore, the interviewee is constrained in terms of mentalizing about (and connecting with) the interviewer. Finally, on an extrapersonal level, *we need to account for mental states of many people at the same time, without any personal interaction.* Thus, we are forced to "average" mental states and verify our assumptions in different ways than we do on an interpersonal level.

AVENUES FOR ENHANCEMENT

By now, you should have a good general understanding of what mentalization entails, and an appreciation of the benefits and challenges associated with this powerful social tool. When we do not have much time or energy, we generally base our inferences about other people on "heuristics" (mental shortcuts and rule-of-thumb strategies that help us make decisions quickly and efficiently) or "stereotypes" (a widely adopted, often unfair and untrue, belief about a particular type of person). This isn't necessarily problematic when it comes to *familiar, straightforward* and *inconsequential* situations. If the situation is *new* or *complex,* however, the chances for misinterpretation and miscalculation increase significantly. In situations such as the court case that we described at the beginning of this chapter, *accurate mentalizing can be a matter of life or death* (literally). We have seen that mentalization encompasses a broad array of competencies. This means that the opportunities for improvement are equally wide-ranging. For instance, people may have gaps in certain fundamental mentalization abilities, or they may have good mentalization skills in general, but they encounter difficulties in employing those skills in particular situations or with particular people.

Mentalization proficiency is associated with a multitude of social and personal advantages. Before we can determine what our mentalization proficiency level is, however, *we need to be able to recognize the indicia of good or poor mentalizing.* This is critical to estimating not only our own level of mentalizing mastery, but also the level of those with whom we interact. Possessing well-developed mentalization skills yourself does not guarantee successful interactions with others, especially those who are struggling with severely *under*developed mentalization skills. As is the case with most social interactions, it takes two to tango. If our interactional counterpart is impaired in their ability to mentalize, social interactions, especially complex ones, can prove to be challenging. Finally, beyond recognizing good or poor mentalizing in others, *we need to be vigilant of the use of tactics that are indicative of pseudomentalization*. Mentalization is our most powerful social tool, and its power invites some people to use tricks that can masquerade as mentalization.

In the remaining chapters of this book, we will provide opportunities for enhancement and refinement of your mentalization skillset culminating in a self-directed learning model for mastering mentalization.

Mentalization Code of Conduct

Finally, because mentalization is our most powerful social tool, a tool that can be used for both good and evil, we have added a "code of conduct" to guide ethical mentalizing behavior. In this code of conduct, we have outlined the social norms and values, responsibilities and practices that should govern responsible mentalization. This code of conduct is comprised of five general principles:

The first principle asserts that:

> We must remain mindful of the influence and the potential consequences that mentalization can have on individuals and groups with whom we deal, and avoid its misuse or abuse at all times.

The second principle stresses that:

> In our dealings with others, we should avoid unjust practices by taking into consideration our biases, our level of mentalization competence and the inherent limitations of mentalization.

The third principle affirms that:

> Our mentalizing efforts should not be done in a way that is viewed by others as misleading, exploitative, or intentionally pernicious.

The fourth principle advocates that:

> At all times, we need to respect the rights and dignity of other people, including their right to privacy and confidentiality.

The fifth and final principle recognizes that:

> Proper mentalization practices should reflect sensitivity to diversity concerns related to such factors as race, ethnicity, gender, religious beliefs, physical or mental disability and socioeconomic status.

Whether you are in the middle of a closing argument, in an important meeting or negotiation, or navigating a difficult conversation, mentalization provides you with the tools you need to survey the social landscape, join forces with others, gain a competitive advantage and achieve your strategic objectives.

References

Apperly, I. (2011). *Mindreaders: the cognitive basis of" theory of mind."* Hove, England: Psychology Press.

Apps, M. A. J., Rushworth, M. F. S., & Chang, S. W. C. (2016). The anterior cingulate gyrus and social cognition: tracking the motivation of others. *Neuron, 90*(4), 692–707. doi:10.1016/j.neuron.2016.04.018

Baron-Cohen, S., Tager-Flusberg, H., & Cohen, D. J. (Eds.). (2013). *Understanding other minds: Perspectives from developmental cognitive neuroscience* (3rd ed.). Oxford University Press.

Basinger, H. & Hogg, J. P. (2020). *Neuroanatomy, Brainstem*. StatPearls Publishing.

Bastiaansen, J. A. C. J., Thioux M., & Keysers C. (2009). Evidence for mirror systems in emotions. *Philosophical Transactions of the Royal Society B: Biological Sciences, 364*(1528), 2391–2404. doi:10.1098/rstb.2009.0058

Bateman, A. W. & Fonagy, P. (2016). *Mentalization-based treatment for personality Disorders: A practical* Guide. Oxford, UK: Oxford University Press ISBN 978-0-19-166992-7.

Brewer, J. A., Worhunsky, P. D., Gray, J. R., Tang, Y.-Y., Weber, J., & Kober, H. (2011). Meditation experience is associated with differences in default mode network activity and connectivity. *Proceedings of the National Academy of Sciences, 108*(50), 20254–20259. doi:10.1073/pnas.1112029108

Brewer, J. A., Garrison, K. A., & Whitfield-Gabrieli, S. (2013). What about the "self" is processed in the posterior cingulate cortex? *Frontiers in Human Neuroscience, 7*(647), 1–7. https://doi.org/10.3389/fnhum.2013.00647

Brewer, J. A., & Garrison, K. A. (2014). The posterior cingulate cortex as a plausible mechanistic target of meditation: findings from neuroimaging. *Annals of the New York Academy of Sciences, 1307*(1), 19–27. doi:10.1111/nyas.12246

Cavanna, A. E., & Trimble, M. R. (2006). The precuneus: a review of its functional anatomy and behavioural correlates. *Brain, 129*(3), 564–583. https://doi.org/10.1093/brain/awl004

Decety, J., Jackson, P. L., Somerville, J. A., Chaminade, T., & Meltzoff, A. N. (2004). The neural bases of cooperation and competition: An fMRI investigation. *NeuroImage, 23*(2), 744-51. doi: 10.1016/j.neuroimage.2004.05.025.

De Waal, F. B. M. (2008). Putting the altruism back into altruism: The evolution of empathy. *Annual Review of Psychology, 59*(1), 279–300. doi:10.1146/annurev.psych.59.103006.093625

Eisenberger, N. I. (2003). Does rejection hurt? An fMRI study of social exclusion. *Science, 302*(5643), 290–292. doi:10.1126/science.1089134

Eslinger, P. J., Moll, J., & de Oliveira-Souza, R. (2001). Emotional and cognitive processing in empathy and moral behavior. *Behavioral and Brain Sciences, 25*(01). doi:10.1017/s0140525x02360011

Fletcher, P.C., Frith, C.D., Baker, S.C., Shallice, T., Frackowiak, R.S.J., & Dolan, R.J. (1995). "The Mind's Eye--Precuneus Activation in Memory-Related Imagery". *NeuroImage, 2* (3): 195–200. doi:10.1006/nimg.1995.1025

Geng, J. J., Vossel, S. (2013). Re-evaluating the role of TPJ in attentional control: Contextual updating? *Neuroscience & Biobehavioral Reviews, 37*(10), 2608–2620. doi:10.1016/j.neubiorev.2013.08.010

Hatfield, E., Cacioppo, J. T., & Rapson, R. L. (1994). *Studies in emotion and social interaction. Emotional contagion*. Cambridge University Press; Editions de la Maison des Sciences de l'Homme.

Hein, G., & Knight, R. T. (2008). Superior temporal sulcus--It's my area: or is it? *Journal of Cognitive Neuroscience, 20*(12), 2125–36. doi: 10.1162/jocn.2008.20148.

Herlin, B., Navarro, V., & Dupont, S., (2021). The temporal pole: From anatomy to function-A literature appraisal. *Journal of Chemical Neuroanatomy, 113*(101925). doi: 10.1016/j.jchemneu.2021.101925.

Hooker, C. I., Verosky, S. C., Germine, L. T., Knight, R. T., & D'Esposito, M. (2008). Mentalizing about emotion and its relationship to empathy. *Social Cognitive and Affective Neuroscience, 3*(3), 204–217. doi: 10.1093/scan/nsn019

Keysers, C., & Gazzola, V. (2006). Towards a unifying neural theory of social cognition. *Progress in Brain Research,* 379–401. doi:10.1016/s0079-6123(06)56021-2

Kinsella, M. T., & Monk, C. (2009). Impact of Maternal Stress, Depression and Anxiety on Fetal Neurobehavioral Development. *Clinical Obstetrics and Gynecology, 52*(3), 425–440. doi:10.1097/grf.0b013e3181b52df1

Laurita, A. C., Hazan, C., & Spreng, R. N. (2019). An attachment theoretical perspective for the neural representation of close others. *Social Cognitive and Affective Neuroscience, 14*(3), 237–251. doi:10.1093/scan/nsz010

Leech, R., Braga, R., & Sharp, D. J. (2012). Echoes of the brain within the posterior cingulate cortex. *Journal of Neuroscience, 32*(1), 215–222. https://doi.org/10.1523/JNEUROSCI.3689-11.2012

Leech, R., & Sharp, D. J. (2014). The role of the posterior cingulate cortex in cognition and disease. *Brain, 137*(1), 12–32. doi:10.1093/brain/awt162

Lieberman, M. D. (2007). Social cognitive neuroscience: A review of core processes. *Annual Review of Psychology, 58*, 259-289. doi:10.1146/annurev.psych.58.110405.085654

Lundstrom, B. N., Ingvar, M., & Petersson, K. M. (2005). The role of precuneus and left inferior frontal cortex during source memory episodic retrieval. *NeuroImage, 27*(4), 824–34. doi:10.1016/j.neuroimage.2005.05.008

Meltzoff, A.N., & Decety, J. (2003). What imitation tells us about social cognition: a rapprochement between developmental psychology and cognitive neuroscience. *Philosophical Transactions of the Royal Society B: Biological Sciences, 358*(1431), 491–500. doi: 10.1098/rstb.2002.1261

Molenberghs, P., Cunnington, R., & Mattingley, J. B. (2009). Is the mirror neuron system involved in imitation? A short review and meta-analysis. *Neuroscience and Biobehavioral Reviews, 33*(7), 975–980. doi:10.1016/j.neubiorev.2009.03.010

Oostenbroek, J., Suddendorf, T., Nielsen, M., Redshaw, J., Kennedy-Costantini, S., Davis, J., Clark, S., & Slaughter, V. (2016). Comprehensive Longitudinal Study Challenges the Existence of Neonatal Imitation in Humans. *Current Biology, 26*(10), 1334–1338. doi:10.1016/j.cub.2016.03.047

Ring, H. A. (2002). Neuropsychiatry of the basal ganglia. *Journal of Neurology, Neurosurgery & Psychiatry, 72*(1), 12–21. doi:10.1136/jnnp.72.1.12

Rizzolatti, G., & Sinigaglia, C. (2008). *Mirrors in the Brain. How We Share our Actions and Emotions.* Oxford (UK), Oxford University Press.

Rubin, R. D., Watson, P. D., Duff, M. C., & Cohen, N. J. (2014). The role of the hippocampus in flexible cognition and social behavior. *Frontiers in Human Neuroscience, 8*(742). doi:10.3389/fnhum.2014.00742

Shahaeian, A., Nielsen, M., Peterson, C. C., Aboutalebi, M., & Slaughter, V. (2014). Knowledge and Belief Understanding Among Iranian and Australian Preschool Children. *Journal of Cross-Cultural Psychology, 45*(10), 1643–1654. doi:10.1177/0022022114548484

Speitel C., Traut-Mattausch, E. & Jonas, E. (2019) Functions of the right DLPFC and right TPJ in proposers and responders in the ultimatum game. *Social Cognitive and Affective Neuroscience, 14*(3), 263–270. https://doi.org/10.1093/scan/nsz005

Spreng, R. N., Mar, R. A., & Kim, A. S. (2009). The common neural basis of autobiographical memory, prospection, navigation, theory of mind, and the default mode: a quantitative meta-analysis. *Journal of Cognitive Neuroscience, 21*(3), 489–510. doi: 10.1162/jocn.2008.21029

Spreng, R. N., & Grady, C. L. (2010). Patterns of brain activity supporting autobiographical memory, prospection, and theory of mind, and their relationship to the default mode network. *Journal of Cognitive Neuroscience, 22*(6), 1112–1123. doi: 10.1162/jocn.2009.21282

Uddin, L. Q., Nomi, J. S., Hébert-Seropian, B., Ghaziri, J., & Boucher, O. (2017). Structure and function of the human insula. *Journal of Clinical Neurophysiology, 34*(4), 300–306. doi:10.1097/wnp.0000000000000377

Van Overwalle, F. (2009). Social cognition and the brain: A meta-analysis. *Human Brain Mapping, 30*(3), 829–858. doi:10.1002/hbm.20547

Van Overwalle, F., Baetens, K., Mariën, P., & Vandekerckhove, M. (2014). Social cognition and the cerebellum: a meta-analysis of over 350 fMRI studies. *NeuroImage, 86*, 554–72. http://doi. org/10.1016/j.neuroimage.2013.09.033.

Wellman, H. M., & Liu, D. (2004). Scaling of theory-of-mind tasks. *Child Development, 75*(2), 523-541. doi:10.2307/3696656

Wellman, H. M., Fang, F., & Peterson, C. C. (2011). Sequential progressions in a theory-of-mind scale: Longitudinal perspectives. *Child Development, 82*(3), 780–792. doi:10.1111/j.1467-8624.2011.01583.x

SECTION II.

BASIC MENTALIZING

To Sense and Perceive

Chapter 1.

Embodied Sharing of Affect and Behavior

Introduction to Basic Mentalizing

Before delving into the particulars of basic mentalizing, we will briefly review the general concept of mentalization at this elementary level. Basic mentalizing pertains to our most primitive level of mentalization. It enables us to read ourselves and others through *non*verbal stimuli, both *internal* (interoceptive) and *external* (exteroceptive), which we generally process without any conscious awareness. We have distinguished three important abilities on this level of mentalization:

1. The ability to detect and identify social signals and cues of others by monitoring changes in our own affect and behavior.
2. The ability to detect social signals and cues in nonverbal behavior that can be used to infer straightforward and immediate mental states that help us explain and predict basic behavior.
3. The ability to recognize the impact of our intero- and exteroceptive sensations on the accuracy of our mental state inferences.

Generally, we are primarily aware of nonverbal social signals and cues that we detect through our visual and auditory information processing channels. There is, however, a vast range of signals and cues that we process unconsciously through basic mentalizing. Becoming aware of our basic mentalizing tendencies helps us to find ways to hone our skills to mentalize on this elementary level. As explained in the previous section, basic mentalizing is *embodied,* i.e., we feel it and act it out. Mentalizing on this level is most often done *unconsciously* and *implicitly*. This level of mentalization *is always online,* meaning that it is always available to us during our interactions with others. Information sharing on this level is *nonverbal, intuitive* and *unplanned*. The advantages of basic mentalizing are that it is *fast, effortless* and *continuous*. The limitations are that it is *primitive, restricted* and *inflexible*. The fact that basic mentalizing is an economical way of mentalizing comes with a trade-off; *the level of accuracy tends to be low in complex situations,* and it is *hard to control*. The primary objectives of mentalizing on this elementary level are:

- To infer people's basic affective mental states and straightforward elemental needs and intentions through their observable nonverbal behavior.

- To connect with others through nonverbal behavior, build rapport and create a positive ambiance so that they do not feel restrained in their nonverbal or verbal behavior.
- To facilitate smooth interaction and elicit prosocial behavior.
- To heighten the accuracy of our higher-level mentalization inferences.
- To stay aware of possible bias in our explanations and predictions of behavior through the monitoring of interoceptive and exteroceptive sensations.
- To be aware of our own inclination to "catch" the affective states of others, or to mimic their behavior.

Being aware of our own susceptibility to affective and behavioral contagion is critical for our understanding that the cause for our feelings, thoughts and behavior can be found within our immediate environment. This understanding helps to lower empathic distress and makes it possible to use this information to draw mental state inferences, or to dissociate from others when we regard their affective states or behavior as unwelcome.

COMPONENTS OF BASIC MENTALIZING

We have divided basic mentalizing into three components:

1. Embodied sharing of affect and behavior
2. Nonverbal social indicator detection
3. Nonsocial sensing and associating

Each component is discussed in a separate chapter. This chapter, *Embodied Sharing of Affect and Behavior,* examines our primitive tendency to share in the affect of others (i.e., their experience of feelings, moods, or emotions) and to synchronize our behavior with people around us. We share affect and behavior through our innate tendencies of mimicry, affective contagion and behavioral contagion. These synchronizing abilities are of critical importance in understanding human cognition, affect and behavior in social interaction. The second chapter, *Nonverbal Social Indicator Detection*, deals with the detection of social indicators that are conveyed nonverbally – such as gestures, postures and facial expressions – without experiencing a strongly embodied sharing. The third chapter, *Nonsocial Sensing and Associating*, pertains to the detection of exteroceptive stimuli (e.g., light intensity or sound amplitude) and interoceptive stimuli (e.g., hunger or fatigue), which can originate independent of social interaction. These indicators might not transmit social information, but they do, nonetheless, have a considerable impact on our attentional focus and our interpretation of social indicators.

The three components of basic mentalizing fit along two spectrums. The first spectrum ranges from *strongly* embodied to *weakly* embodied in relation to our sensorial responses. In other words, these are things that we feel ourselves versus things that we are aware of but do not feel ourselves. Embodied sharing of affect and behavior and nonsocial sensing and associating are strongly embodied indicator gathering systems, while nonverbal social indicators are gathered through observation and are not "felt" as such. The second spectrum runs from *social* indicator detection to *nonsocial* indicator detection. Embodied sharing of affect and behavior and nonverbal social indicators predominantly transmit signals and cues that result from social interaction, while nonsocial sensations are generally independent of social interaction. The latter are brought about by unrelated internal changes in our body, or by situational and environmental causes such as the weather or context. We will now examine the first component of basic mentalizing: Embodied Sharing of Affect and Behavior.

Mass Psychogenic Illness

In the late summer of 2011, a number of teenage students at the LeRoy Junior-Senior High School in the town of Leroy, New York, began to exhibit unexplained medical symptoms similar to those seen in "tourette syndrome" (repetitive verbal outbursts, speech difficulties, facial tics, muscle seizures, etc.). In January 2012, public health authorities determined that the students were suffering from "conversion disorder," a mental condition in which a person experiences blindness, paralysis, or other neurological symptoms without a known physical origin. Officials could not identify an environmental cause for the behavior, and suggested that perhaps social media had helped to spread the so-called "infection." One factor that pointed to a probable psychological cause was the fact that the individuals who posted their symptoms on Facebook recovered more slowly than those who did not communicate publicly about their ailments. This phenomenon is known as "mass psychogenic illness." The online *APA* (American Psychology Association) *Dictionary of Psychology (2022),* defines "psychogenic" as "resulting from mental factors." The dictionary goes on to say: "The term is used particularly to denote or refer to a disorder that cannot be accounted for by any identifiable physical dysfunction and is believed to be due to psychological factors (e.g., a conversion disorder)."

Mass psychogenic illness involves the appearance of symptoms spread throughout a group of people, or even throughout an entire population. While these symptoms are real, there is no evidence that they are produced by an external cause such as a virus or environmental pollution. Mass psychogenic illness is not a new phenomenon. In fact, it is quite common when you look at historical events. For instance, beginning in the Middle Ages and extending into the 17th century, a social phenomenon called "dancing mania," also known as "dancing plague" or "choreomania," spread across Europe. Large groups of people, sometimes numbering in the hundreds, would spontaneously and uncontrollably dance and jump together, with members occasionally succumbing to heart attack, stroke, or some other self-inflicted injury. You can find many more examples of mass psychogenic illness throughout the centuries. Mass psychogenic illness remains a controversial phenomenon, as it is difficult to explain the symptoms purely in terms of psychological factors. Some researchers have hypothesized that its cause might be due to extreme stress, while others have suggested that some people are just very susceptible to affective and behavioral contagion. A number of scientists believe that mass psychogenic illness is a real phenomenon and that it can afflict anybody if certain critical factors line up. These historical events are extreme examples of affective and behavioral contagion. More common, and less severe, examples are found in various studies on the subject. Interestingly, these studies demonstrate that we get "infected" not only by audiovisual signals, but also via smell. To illustrate, an airline passenger who suffers from a fear of flying may give off a scent of fear that causes other passengers seated in the same area to feel anxious or nervous themselves, even though they normally feel at ease when flying. As demonstrated by these examples, the sharing of affect and behavior, while critical to mentalization, can also work against us.

Embodied sharing of affect and behavior concerns the primitive tendency to synchronize our affect and behavior with our social environment. This sharing of affect and behavior with others is brought about through mimicry, and the associated conveyance of affect and behavior - also referred to as affective and behavioral contagion. Historical events relating to mass psychogenic illness give us a sense of how powerful affective and behavioral contagion can be.

The sharing of experiences through mimicry, affective contagion and behavioral contagion provides a starting point for the recognition of mental states, and helps us to form connections with others. Affect and behavior are often shared subconsciously. At a subconscious level, the tendency to synchronize affect and behavior does *not involve any differentiation between self and others*. In other words, we experience the shared affect and behavior as though they originated within ourselves. This can lead to confusion, since we do not automatically consider the possibility that our own affects and behaviors actually originated with others. When we are not aware of this third-party influence, we miss the opportunity to gain insight into the mental states of others. On the other hand, if we are aware of this tendency, we can regulate the degree to which we are influenced by it. We are able to separate our own affects and behaviors from those of others, and mentalize more effectively about others. Let us take a look at what mimicry, affective contagion and behavioral contagion entail.

Mimicry

"Mimicry" is the action or skill of imitating someone or something. It covers a wide spectrum of different reactions (facial, verbal, emotional and behavioral) through which we imitate others. We mimic others predominantly through our personal interactions with them. We can, however, also mimic others as a result of looking at a picture of them. The imitative behavior of mimicry facilitates the learning of new behaviors and skills from others. Moreover, it helps to strengthen our connection with others, as it is done, for the most part, with affiliative intent. Most important, mimicry functions as a source of social information from which we can infer mental states.

The tendency of humans to mimic one another comes naturally, as it is rooted in our neurophysiological evolution. Often, we are not even conscious of the tendency. Studies show that mimicry is strongly associated with success in social interaction that relies on "synchronization of actions." In a sense, through mimicry we become more "similar" to others in how we feel and act, and this provides us with the opportunity to read others by *examining our own feelings and behaviors*. "Affective mimicry," although not itself a form of empathy, has been associated with empathic accuracy when people consciously use their "mimicked" internal state as a source of information with regard to the affective mental states of others. Becoming more aware of the mimicking behavior of other people is further instructive in understanding the relationships between people in general, and understanding our own interpersonal relationships. Mimicry helps us to strengthen existing relationships and to foster new connections with others. The absence of mimicking behavior, on the other hand, promotes social distancing. It can communicate a higher level of self-esteem, a sense of independence, or dominance over another. It is important, however, to be aware of the costs associated with mimicking others. Studies have shown that when a person is not honest about the way he or she feels, the mimicker tends to infer the affective mental state of the mimickee from the dishonest display. Additionally, these studies found that a mimicker was less able to detect a deceptive emotional display than a person was who did not mimic the other (Stel et al., 2009). Studies suggest that mimicking can lower the mimickee's self-liking, and consequently their self-esteem, making them more inclined, for instance, to apply impression management to regain self-liking. This dynamic has been associated with the tendency for dishonest self-disclosure in, for instance, psychotherapy (see Stel et al., 2009; Muniak et al., 2021). Other research suggests that mimicry can elicit stereotypical behavior in the person who is being mimicked. This seems to occur when people who are being mimicked perceive others as expecting them to display such behavior. The mimicker, in turn, will be more exposed to stereotypical behavior confirming the mimicker's beliefs in stereotypes (Leander et al., 2011).

There are situations where two or more people display the same emotion or behavior, but not on account of mimicry. For instance, when two or more people witness a car accident, they may experience the same emotion (distress) and act in the same way (interrupt what they were doing and focus on the accident), a "parallel elicitation" of affect and behavior rather than a form of mimicry. Alternatively, a person may use the emotional or behavioral expression of another person as a guide for appropriate action in a particular social situation, a mechanism known as "social referencing." The term "mirroring" (the exact copying of another's affective expression or behavior) is often used interchangeably with mimicry, but mirroring does not encompass the full breadth of mimicry. Mimicry, unlike mirroring, can include variations of the original behavior. Mimicry is sometimes purposely exaggerated and used as a form of ridicule. Although the differences between mimicry and mirroring are minor, studies have shown that mirrored mimicry is more conducive to connecting with others than *non*-mirrored mimicry. Mimicry, regardless whether it is mirrored or non-mirrored, can on the other hand, make the person who is mimicked feel uneasy. Thus, when using mimicry as a tactic to connect with others, a technique sometimes taught in training on nonverbal behavior, it is important to *appropriately modulate the degree of imitation and seamlessly match the demands of the social situation*, something that is easier said than done. Most people can readily detect when the mimicking of their affective state or behavior by others does not come naturally. There are, however, practices that can help to promote our natural tendency to mimic others. To illustrate, a high level of attentional focus on the behavior of others together with a genuine interest in their mental states can elicit natural mimicking behavior. When mimicking others, it is equally important to *select the right type of behavior to mimic*. For instance, you should mimic behavior that helps you connect with the other person rather than behavior that can be inferred as social distancing, such as crossing your arms in front of your chest when the other person exhibits the same defensive gesture. It goes without saying that one should never mimic a person's unique expressions due to, for instance, a dialect or a speech impediment.

Conscious mirroring can serve an important function as well. For instance, "parental" mirroring of an infant's expressions, if done in an appropriate way, is considered a critical, intuitive parenting response, essential for the development of a secure attachment relationship between caregivers and infants. Moreover, it facilitates the infant's development of a healthy sense of self and good self-regulation abilities. Mimicry does not necessarily lead to the shared subjective state of mind present with affective contagion, as we will discuss in the next paragraph.

Affective Contagion

"Affective contagion" is *a form of social contagion* involving the spontaneous embodiment of emotions and related behaviors of others. It often starts with mimicry, followed by sensory feedback via our interoceptive system that associates the most likely affect to the behavior. "Interoception" is the perception of stimuli coming from within the body such as heart palpitations, hunger, or stomachache. Interoceptive sensitivity, awareness and accuracy in social situations can be referred to as "social interoception" (Arnold et al., 2019). The process of social interoception has a predictive component as the gathering of social signals and cues through our sensory feedback adds significant power to our ability to infer mental states. This aspect of social interoception is described by Barrett et al. (2016) as "predictive interoceptive coding." Unlike the temporary behavioral response associated with mimicry, the emotion, feeling, or mood elicited by affective contagion can persist even *after* the triggering event has passed. Moreover, the same affect can *resurface* if we later find ourselves in similar circumstances. With affective contagion, affects are transferred not only by direct interaction with, and observation of, other people, as is the case with mimicry, but also via third-party accounts, or triggered memories of an event. Affective states can also be transmitted by music, pictures, or movies. Affective contagion can manifest itself in two ways: first, as a "similar response" – for example, aggression by one person triggers aggression in another, and second, as a "complementary response" – for example, the display of anger by one person triggers a fearful response in another. *The potential for alternate responses* illustrates another key difference between mimicry and affective contagion. Like mimicry, affective contagion is so prevalent in our social environment that it provides valuable fodder for mentalizing, particularly when it comes to recognizing affective states. Affective contagion may even be superior to mimicry in facilitating emotion recognition, as it actually leads to a shared subjective state. Hatfield et al. (1994) even went so far as to propose that "to gain the best insight into another person's affective state one might better focus on one's own feelings than to try to infer it via reasoning." Next, we explore behavioral contagion.

Behavioral Contagion

"Behavioral contagion" is the *subconscious, spontaneous, unsolicited* and *uncritical* adoption of the behavior of other people. Similar to affective contagion, it is often elicited through mimicry, and the effects can last well beyond the triggering behavior. As with affective contagion, behaviors are transferred not only by direct interaction with other people, but also via third-party accounts or depictions, or triggered memories of an event. Even putting on clothes that have a particular social meaning, such as a police officer's uniform, can make a person behave (and feel) in a manner consistent with someone who needs to wear such attire for work. As depicted in our earlier example of mass psychogenic illness, behavioral contagion can operate as a powerful social influence. Adopting the communication style of a person you admire when addressing others is another example of behavioral contagion. Analogous to affective contagion, behavioral contagion can influence a person to display *similar* behavioral patterns, or *complementary* (opposite) behavioral patterns. For instance, dressing in a certain way may induce a similar clothing style preference in others that "infectiously" spreads through the population. Alternatively, when one party dresses in a certain way, the other party may choose to accentuate a different clothing style preference as a reaction to the other. This is an example of a complementary response. When dealing with someone we dislike, our natural inclination is to behave in a complementary way so as to socially distance ourselves from them. Behavior that we adopt through behavioral contagion often informs others about mental states that are linked to these behaviors, such as a particular belief indicated by the rituals of others that we imitate.

Factors That Influence Our Tendency to Share in Affect and Behavior

Our tendency for mimicry, affective contagion and behavioral contagion can be elucidated in intrapersonal, interpersonal and extrapersonal terms. On the intrapersonal level, research indicates that a multitude of factors can impact our tendency to share in the affect and behavior of others. *Experiences in early life* can make us predisposed to be highly responsive to affective and behavioral contagion, or leave us virtually impervious to it. To illustrate, children may be especially sensitive to the changing moods of a troubled parent due to anxiety about their own safety. Our *temperament, personality* and *self-construals,* and our more *transient mental states* are additional important factors. More outgoing and expressive individuals tend to be better transmitters, or more successful at influencing others to feel what they feel and behave in the way they behave. People who have little interest in others, or who are temporarily preoccupied with their own problems or negative emotions, are less likely to pick up on or copy the affects or behaviors of others. A happy mood, on the other hand, heightens the tendency to mimic others. In regard to self-construals, individuals who see themselves as *interdependent* or *dependent* are more inclined to mimic others than are individuals who view themselves as *independent.* People who view themselves as inferior are more inclined to absorb the affect, and copy the behavior, of the people whom they hold in high esteem.

On the interpersonal level, studies reveal that our motivation to mimic others depends on the *person with whom we are dealing*. We are especially likely to mimic those about whom we care, for instance, friends and family members. Mothers are particularly prone to share the emotions of their infant children. On the other hand, it is difficult to share the emotions or behavior of someone whom we dislike. In fact, we may tend to exhibit complementary or contrary emotions or behavior with such people. Another interpersonal factor that can influence our tendency for mimicry, affective contagion and behavioral contagion is *similarity*. We are more inclined to mimic others with whom we share similarities, for instance, a common religious affiliation or social background. People of the same gender also take on the emotions and behaviors of each other more readily. The *nature of the relationship* we have with others is another important factor. Professionals, such as psychotherapists, who have a psychological investment in the welfare of their patients, are more vulnerable to contagion. Research shows that a person of lower status tends to mimic a person of higher status more readily than the other way around. When people find themselves in a leadership position, a heightened sense of responsibility with regard to the well-being or performance of their subordinates can, however, increase their own level of affective and behavioral contagion toward their subordinates. If we admire others, or think of them as more powerful, we are more likely to become "infected" by the way they feel and behave. Conversely, we are less likely to mimic someone to whom we attribute negative characteristics, since our imitation of them would be viewed as "dysfunctional." Also, we do not tend to mimic emotions and behavior that are contrary to our own state of mind. For instance, we are not likely to share a victory dance with our competitors when they prevail over us.

On an extrapersonal level, there are two principal factors that influence our tendency for affective and behavioral mimicry and contagion. The first is *culture*. People from western cultures demonstrate less susceptibility to being "infected" than their eastern counterparts, as more than one study has shown. This variation might be due, in part, to cultural differences in self construal, with westerners generally seeing themselves as *in*dependent and easterners as *inter*dependent. Cultural differences in attitudes toward affective expression and distinct behavioral customs can account for disparities in the tendency to spontaneously share in affective states and behavior. Still, some unfamiliar behaviors, such as "the Indian head shake," can be very contagious. The second factor is *context*. Context can invite the copying of affect and behavior, for example, in the area of artistic expression (dance or sing-along). Likewise, mutually experiencing a disturbing event can make people more inclined to copy each other's affect and behavior reflexively. An angry mob can elicit anger, sometimes even mob behavior, in bystanders. In any social interaction, clearly expressed feelings and goals can exert a powerful influence on the direction and character of affective and behavioral contagion. By contrast, situations in which people have distinct roles to play, and the copying of behavior would impede a desired outcome, considerably lower the tendency to share in affect and behavior. Similarly, when we see other people breaking the rules, our strong belief in playing by the rules may prevent us from following their lead.

We will now examine the key advantages of understanding the human tendency to share affect and behavior.

Understanding Embodied Sharing of Affect and Behavior: Advantages, Impediments and Avenues for Enhancement

ADVANTAGES

There are several key advantages to understanding the human tendency to share in the affect and behavior of others, and to applying this knowledge in everyday life. On an intrapersonal level, *we gain better control over our own inclinations to mimic others.* For example, when we feel insecure, we may become more susceptible to the affective and behavioral influences of others. Learning to regulate our own mental states can be vital to avoiding emotional depletion or fatigue due to the sharing of the affects and behaviors of others.

On an interpersonal level, awareness of our human tendency to share in the affect and behavior of others *facilitates mentalizing about them through the examination of our own feelings and behavior*. Understanding our tendency to imitate others helps us to distinguish our own sensations and behavioral inclinations from those that we "catch" from others. This is important as it helps us to identify the cause of our own unwanted affects and behaviors, and to implement corrective measures at the right source.

Additionally, awareness of this synchronizing tendency enables us to assess whether others want to affiliate with us, to form or solidify connections with others, to learn from and about others and/or to cooperate more effectively with others. It also makes us better equipped to socially distance ourselves from others in subtle ways by ignoring or opposing their behavior. Furthermore, it enables us to more quickly and accurately recognize relationships between people – who enjoys superior status, who likes/dislikes whom, who the decision maker is, etc. In the interactions that we have with others in a group setting we can detect valuable information by observing people who are not at the center of attention and gauging their mental states. For instance, during negotiations we can learn a great deal by paying attention to how ancillary members of the opposing negotiating team behave, even as their lead negotiator masterfully maintains a poker face. Finally, *we can elicit behavioral change in others*, in a nonverbal and non-confrontational way, by "infecting" others with our own displays of the desired behavior or affect.

On an extrapersonal level, our understanding of the human tendency to share in affect and behavior *enables us to be more adept at detecting and resisting covert social influences* that target our affective mental states and behavior on a subconscious level, "inoculating" us against groupthink and mindless conformity. The recognition that people around us influence our affect and behavior enables us to choose work and living environments that match our psychophysiological makeup. Additionally, *it enables us to identify sociocultural differences in affective displays and other behavior* as a potential rationale for our reluctance to synchronize with unfamiliar behavior. This intercultural perceptiveness bolsters our understanding of how these sociocultural differences can impact social interaction.

IMPEDIMENTS

There are a number of factors that impede the ability to use our knowledge of the human tendency to share in the affect and behavior of others to our advantage. As we have seen, *our sharing of affect and behavior remains largely below our level of consciousness*. This presents a major intrapersonal challenge, as it can lead to unexplained stress and negative feelings. It can also lead us to behave in a way that does not align with our own values and beliefs. If we remain unconscious of these affective and behavioral influences, we overlook or misinterpret many interesting and telling social signals and cues, which can obstruct our judgment. Another challenge on the intrapersonal level is *achieving the right balance of sensitivity*. If we are too susceptible to the moods and behaviors of others, social encounters can become confusing and exhausting. If we are not sensitive enough to affective or behavioral contagion and its effects, we fail to detect signals and cues that help to guide socially appropriate behavior, making us more vulnerable to committing "social faux pas" (social blunders or breaches of etiquette, embarrassing or insulting behavior, etc.).

Interpersonally, *the inability to maintain a "proper self-other distinction"* can present a difficult challenge. When we suffer from a "diffused self-other distinction," we assume that the affect we feel or the way we behave has originated within ourselves. We do not realize how much we are influenced by the affect and behavior of people around us. To illustrate, a person may hyperventilate when exposed to the stress or anxiety of others. If people do not consider affective contagion as a potential cause for their physical distress, they could easily relate it to a possible heart attack or another source of anxiety.

On an extrapersonal level, we have learned from the historical accounts of mass psychogenic illness how powerful the sharing of group affect and behavior can be. *It can "infect" large numbers of people to the point of social disruption.* We may assume that being infected by positive feelings and behavior is always a good thing, but this is not universally true. Just consider the behavior of people at an art auction. The excitement generated by the competitive bidding process surrounding that one unique masterpiece has led to more than one case of buyer's remorse for the so-called "successful" bidder. The power of shared affect and behavior is routinely used by larger entities such as governments or organizations to influence crowds to their benefit. With regard to context, *we are easily influenced, both affectively and behaviorally, by sensory aspects* such as pictures, symbols, or music that "infect" us with the impression that they make on us. Architects specializing in aural architecture, for instance, are well aware of how the audible aspects of spaces can produce an affective and behavioral response in people. *Conscious* basic mentalizing helps us to become more aware of what is happening around us, which gives us the opportunity to control and arrest the "contagion" if it is unwanted.

AVENUES FOR ENHANCEMENT

By now, you should have a good understanding of what the embodied sharing of affect and behavior entails, and an appreciation of the benefits and challenges associated with this aspect of basic mentalizing. We would like to conclude this chapter by offering some suggestions and opportunities for enhancing your understanding of this human tendency, and applying your newfound knowledge in everyday life. The first step is to *conduct a self-assessment* to determine where you fit on the embodied sharing susceptibility spectrum (in other words, your inclination to "catch" the affects and mimic the behavior of others). Once you have established a baseline, you can use it to detect and regulate your sensitivity to this type of influence. The second step is to *understand and actively engage in the embodied sharing process*, as this will facilitate affective and cognitive self-regulation. Here, the focus should be on achieving a healthy self-other distinction. The third step is to *enhance your ability to detect relevant embodied signals and cues in yourself and others* to make meaningful inferences in support of your higher-level mentalizing activities.

References

American Psychological Association. (n.d.). Psychogenic. In *APA dictionary of psychology*. Retrieved July 17, 2022, from https://dictionary.apa.org/psychogenic

Arnold, A. J., Winkielman P., & Dobkins, K. (2019). Interoception and social connection. *Frontiers in Psychology, 10*(2589). doi: 10.3389/fpsyg.2019.02589

Barrett, L. F., Quigley, K. S., & Hamilton, P. (2016). An active inference theory of allostasis and interoception in depression. *Philosophical Transactions of the*

Royal Society B: Biological Sciences, 371(1708). doi:https://doi.org/10.1098/rstb.2016.0011

Hatfield, E., Cacioppo, J. T., & Rapson, R. L. (1994). *Studies in emotion and social interaction. Emotional contagion*. Cambridge University Press; Editions de la Maison des Sciences de l'Homme.

Leander, N. P., Chartrand, T. L., & Wood, W. (2011). Mind your mannerisms: Behavioral mimicry elicits stereotype conformity. *Journal of Experimental Social Psychology, 47*(1), 195–201. https://doi.org/10.1016/j.jesp.2010.09.002

Muniak, P., Dolinski, D., Grzyb, T., Cantarero. K., & Kulesza, W. (2021) You Want to Know the Truth? Then Don't Mimic! The Link Between Mimicry and Lying. Zeitschrift für Psychologie, 229(3), 185–190. https://doi.org/10.1027/2151-2604/a000451

Stel, M., van Dijk, E., Olivier, E. (2009). You Want to Know the Truth? Then Don't Mimic! *Psychological Science, 20*(6), 693–699. doi:10.1111/j.1467-9280.2009.02350.x

SECTION II.

BASIC MENTALIZING

To Sense and Perceive

Chapter 2.

Nonverbal Social Indicator Detection

Cold Reading

There are people who claim to possess powers that enable them to mysteriously read your mind, or to provide insights into your life and your future. Some even go as far as claiming that they can make contact with your dead relatives. Despite their assertions, the existence of such powers has not been substantiated by scientific data. The most common method employed by such charlatans is known as "cold reading." Cold reading illustrates how powerfully nonverbal behavior can be used by illusionists, psychics and others to trick us into believing that they have supernatural mindreading powers. Cold reading is a form of pseudomentalization whereby the so-called "mentalist" implies that he knows much more about us than he actually does. Through the use of observable information such as age, gender and/or ethnic origin, these mentalists make assumptions and engage in high-probability guesswork about their human subject, all the while judging the subject's nonverbal reactions to gauge whether they are on the right track. They follow up not only on the subject's verbal responses, but particularly on promising nonverbal reactions of the subject, to emphasize and reinforce possible new connections. This technique is known as "shotgunning," as it relies upon a wide pattern of "projectiles" to increase the likelihood of "hitting the mark." These practices seem to work due to "confirmation bias" - our tendency to gather evidence that confirms preexisting expectations. The success of these tactics is also attributable to the "Barnum effect," also called the "Forer effect," which is defined in the *APA Dictionary of Psychology* (2022) as "[t]he tendency to believe that vague predictions or general personality descriptions, such as those offered by astrology, have specific applications to oneself." For instance, using the cold reading method, the mentalist utters the following line, "*I sense that you are sometimes insecure.*" Because we all feel insecure at times, it is easy for the subject to affirm such a statement. Beyond cold reading, mentalists often employ a method known as "warm reading," which involves the judicious use of the aforementioned Barnum effect. Yet another technique employed by mentalists is "hot-reading," which couples either or both of the foregoing measures with information gathered through background research or eavesdropping.

Cold reading is considered pseudomentalization, as the aim of the mentalist is not really to gain the perspective of the subject. In fact, they are not at all interested in the subject's mental states. Cold readers use this information to *shape* the perspective of their subject rather than trying to gain insight into the subject's point of view. Psychics, illusionists, and sometimes clergy or negotiators, who rely on these tactics, are merely trying to impress us through clever manipulation of our behavior. In addition, they employ their own nonverbal behavior to appear confident, to seem modest about their ability, and to engender our cooperation by telling us that the more fully we participate, the better their reading, counsel, or negotiation outcome will be. These manipulative behaviors work together to gradually lower our critical reasoning skills and pave the way for unquestioning belief and willing collaboration. Such so-called "mentalists" can be so convincing that we start to believe in the pseudo reality that they propose. People who feel vulnerable or desperately hope to see a particular outcome – such as locating a missing person - are especially susceptible to these practices. In a well-publicized account, British entrepreneur Naill Rice spent approximately 460,000 British Pounds on psychics with the aim of winning back his lover, all to no avail. Cold reading is not always employed for dishonest purposes. It can also be used as a form of entertainment by popular illusionists who play innocent tricks with our minds.

This second chapter on basic mentalizing deals with the detection of social indicators that are conveyed *nonverbally* – such as gestures, postures and facial expressions - *without the embodied sharing* that accompanies mimicry, affective contagion and behavioral contagion. These nonverbal social indicators can be "extralinguistic," in other words not involving, or beyond the bounds of, verbal communication (e.g., hand gestures). Alternatively, they can be "paralinguistic," which pertains to the non-lexical elements of speech, for example, tone of voice. In popular literature, nonverbal behavior is often referred to as "body language." Nonverbal behavior is, however, broader in scope than body language, as it also encompasses other expressive aspects, such as the way we decorate our house to make an impression. The use of emoticons in electronic communications is a recently appearing form of nonverbal behavior.

The subject matter of this chapter pertains to the observation and interpretation of social indicators on a level that does not require the embodied sharing that is always present with mimicry, affective contagion and behavioral contagion. What do we mean by nonverbal social indicator detection? Nonverbal social indicator detection concerns our ability to infer social information from observable affective and intent mental state indicators:

- via physical signals and cues,
- via the sensory environment we create to give people an impression of ourselves, and
- via the way we choose to interact with others on a nonverbal level.

While the social indicators that we display via our physical appearance reveal information about our identity, background and personality, the way we *choose* to interact with others reveals social information about our interpersonal relationships, and our perceptions of the world around us. Why are nonverbal indicators so important in relation to mentalization?

The Importance of Nonverbal Social Indicators

Nonverbal social signals and cues provide valuable information about *social rules, affective states* or *intentions*. They function to bring about a response – influencing people to either *act* or to *refrain from acting*. There are three aspects of nonverbal indicator detection that we need to keep in mind:

1. Nonverbal social signals and cues are discernible behaviors that people exhibit during social interaction.
2. These social indicators produce changes in our mental states or in the mental states of others.
3. These changes in mental states are not random, but follow principles and laws of human behavior. This is precisely why we are able to use this information to predict or explain behavior.

Nonverbal communication is a major part of the human interaction and communication process. It is often claimed that more than 90% of all meaning comes from nonverbal indicators. This would suggest that less than 10% of meaning would come from verbal content. As research shows, however, this is unlikely, since there are many circumstances in which spoken dialogue carries far more weight than nonverbal behavior. Nonetheless, it cannot be disputed that nonverbal indicators contribute significantly to our social interactions. Interestingly, studies have shown that when verbal messages contradict nonverbal ones, we tend to believe the nonverbal messages over the verbal ones. These findings illustrate our reliance on the decoding of nonverbal signals and cues in our search for another person's mental states.

The most obvious function of nonverbal communication is message production and processing, but scholars have proposed a variety of additional functions that nonverbal behaviors serve. For instance, nonverbal communication can *clarify*, *strengthen* or *attenuate* our affective and verbal expressions. Additionally, it facilitates social cognition, enabling us to better navigate the waters of social interaction. It also plays an important role in impression formation, enabling us to display either a true or desired identity, or to assume the guise of a character in a play. It turns out that we rely much more on nonverbal behavior than on verbal behavior to gauge the feelings or attitudes of others. This should come as no surprise, since affect is largely conveyed via observable indicators, and attitudes have a significant affective component. Furthermore, we apply nonverbal behavior to connect with others, to manage our conversations and to communicate relational messages.

Why is nonverbal communication so influential? First of all, *it is ubiquitous*. Every action or inaction has the capacity to convey meaning. Moreover, *it is multifunctional*. A variety of different nonverbal channels can be used in parallel. From an evolutionary standpoint, nonverbal communication emerged earlier in human development than spoken language. Similarly, from the time we are born, we start using nonverbal behavior, well before we begin to use language. Sometimes, nonverbal communication is the only available means of communication. For instance, when we are in a foreign country and do not speak the local language, we often revert to nonverbal communication to facilitate mutual understanding, although this can sometimes actually lead to confusion, as the same gesture can have different meanings from one culture to the next. Nonverbal behavior also facilitates task understanding and goal directedness. And finally, nonverbal communication can be used to deceive others, and at the same time, to guard against acts of deception.

The Relationship Between Verbal and Nonverbal Social Indicators

At the basic mentalizing level we focus on nonverbal communication. It can be instructive, however, to take a moment to examine the ways in which verbal and nonverbal communication work together. Understanding this dynamic can help us to better identify what to look for when it comes to mental state indicators, and how to interpret these pieces of meaningful data. When we meet others, nonverbal behavior generally precedes verbal behavior, and therefore provides the initial social information upon which we form a first impression. At times, nonverbal communication is the best (or the only) way that we have to express ourselves. For instance, when we find it emotionally difficult to speak, or when we can't speak at all due to an impairment, injury, or trauma, we can generally still resort to nonverbal communication. Sometimes nonverbal communication is more appropriate than its verbal counterpart. This can be observed in ceremonial acts, such as bowing or saluting. Nonverbal behavior can be necessary when we do not want people to take us literally, for example, when we are joking or using sarcasm. Verbal and nonverbal behavior can complement one another. While verbal communication is essentially a *sequential* process, nonverbal communication channels can *operate in parallel*. For instance, I can tell you that I don't have time to talk to you while letting out a sigh and simultaneously looking at my watch. When we allow verbal and nonverbal behavior to work together, we can "fine-tune" our messages to fit situational demands. We can strengthen, clarify, or soften our message as required by the circumstances. On the other hand, when a person's verbal and nonverbal communications do not appear to align, it can be a sign of intrapersonal confusion, or internal conflict, that the person is struggling with or is trying to hide. We see this often in "mixed-motive situations" in which one or more of the parties are faced with a conflict between the motive to affiliate/cooperate and the motive to dissociate/compete, for instance, when colleagues need to work together but at the same time are in competition for the same promotion. A perceived mismatch between nonverbal and verbal behavior can, however, also be due to our own misconception of how a person should behave in relation to the verbal message they are expressing. Therefore, it is important not to jump to conclusions when interpreting perceived inconsistencies. The ability to detect and decode such inconsistencies is a critical basic mentalizing skill, as it helps us to understand when we need to seek further clarification. We all communicate in complex ways, relying on a multitude of mental faculties to *encode* and *decode* social messages. Some of our nonverbal communication faculties, such as basic emotional expressions, are *innate* and *based on biological characteristics* (although even these expressions are subject to cultural influences). Other nonverbal communication faculties, such as shaking hands or bowing upon greeting another person, are *acquired,* and *adjusted* to the social and cultural environment. We all use a combination of these biological and acquired encoding/decoding processes to produce and interpret social signals and cues. The biological and sociocultural processes involved in producing and interpreting social signals often operate *independently.* For instance, some affective facial expressions result primarily from nervous system arousal, while others are more attributable to conditioned responses, e.g., a genuine smile versus a smile out of politeness. Innate encoding mechanisms produce nonverbal messages that are easier to decode than those shaped by sociocultural influences. To decode the latter, we need to take underlying sociocultural factors into consideration.

Nonverbal Social Indicator Conveyors

What kinds of nonverbal social indicators can we observe in others? We use various senses to detect nonverbal signals and cues, including our powers of auditory and visual perception and our sense of smell and touch. Let us examine the different means people use to convey nonverbal social indicators.

"**Kinesics**" is an important category of nonverbal behavior whereby we derive meaningful communication through the interpretation of physical expressions. The term kinesics was first used in 1952 by anthropologist Ray Birdwhistell, who studied how people communicate through posture, gesture, stance and movement. Kinesics convey information, the interpretation of which varies depending on the sociocultural setting. Birdwhistell pointed out that "human gestures differ from those of other animals in that they are polysemic, that they can be interpreted to have many different meanings depending on the communicative context in which they are produced." He also resisted the idea that "'body language' could be deciphered in some absolute fashion." He further proposed that "every body movement must be interpreted broadly and in conjunction with every other element in communication." Let us take a look at the different types of body movement, starting with gestures.

"**Gestures**" are movements of a part of the body – especially movements of the hand or head - used to communicate an idea or meaning. A gesture can communicate meaning on its own, or it can be used to clarify and guide verbal communication. Examples include:

- "**Emblems**," which are gestures with a symbolic meaning that require no further explanation, for example, waving at someone to say "hello."
- "**Regulators**," which are gestures that help maintain or regulate turn-taking, such as conversational gestures, for instance, nodding your head to encourage someone to continue speaking.

- "**Illustrators**" (or gesticulations), which are kinesics that help to clarify and influence the quality of a verbal message, such as stretching your hands apart when describing something as being big.

"**Adaptors**," also known as manipulators, are nonverbal social indicators that satisfy physical or psychological needs, for instance, to lower levels of anxiety or reduce discomfort. Adaptors are body movements whereby we use one body part to manipulate another body part (or an object) to make ourselves feel more comfortable. Self-adaptors are movements that most often involve self-touch, such as scratching or stroking one's hair. Adaptors are not usually intended as communications, and thus they function more often as cues instead of signals. They do, however, reveal mental states, and are sometimes used to communicate disrespect, such as leaning back and putting one's feet on the office desk. Consequently, adaptors can be instructive for mentalization.

"**Body posture**" provides another way for human beings to display their mental states nonverbally. In addition, body posture can indicate the strength of mental states like affects, desires and beliefs. It can also reveal intent. For instance, if we want to convince others of our belief, we show confidence and a sense of urgency through the way we speak, sit, or stand. Or, when listening intently to the narrative of another, we sit or stand in a way that invites the other to disclose more. Body posture and movement are, however, prone to misinterpretation. To illustrate, covering your mouth could be taken by another person as suppression of emotion and perhaps uncertainty. It could, however, actually signify that you are thinking hard or are unsure of what to say next.

Another category of kinesics is "**facial expressions**," the most recognizable means we have of physically expressing emotions in order to communicate with and influence our surroundings, to elicit behaviors in others, such as receiving assistance, or to discourage unwelcome behavior. Combinations of facial movements involving the eyes (and the area surrounding the eyes, including the eyebrows), the lips, the nose and the cheeks, communicate different messages. Facial expressions can indicate affective mental states such as emotions (happiness, anger, sadness), moods (romantic, optimistic, depressed) and feelings (fatigue, discomfort, irritation, confusion). Nonverbal expressions of basic emotions, such as sadness and anger, are generally unambiguous, and therefore less susceptible to misinterpretation. The brain seems to process facial expression and body posture in conjunction with each other. Recognition of affect and intent indicators is significantly enhanced when facial expressions are accompanied by complementary body posture and movement. To illustrate, when people show anger, they may feel stronger, they often display a dominant body posture, and their body movements show approach tendencies. When people are fearful, on the other hand, they may feel weaker, they often display a submissive body posture, and their body movements display avoidance tendencies. Facial expressions, along with other accompanying kinesics, do more than simply demonstrating affects or intent. They also indicate other mental states, such as disbelief, interest, reflectiveness, intention, etc. They change dynamically in consonance with mental states and social action (including the consideration of social display rules or the desire to hide true feelings).

"**Oculesics**," considered by many to be a subcategory of kinesics, is the study of eye contact, movement and behavior as a form of nonverbal communication. Oculesics pertains to nonverbal communication focusing on the derivation of meaning from eye behavior. The length, direction, duration and reciprocation of a person's gaze can be very informative. Joint attention, i.e., looking at the same thing another person is looking at, is viewed as one of the hallmarks of visual perspective taking, which is a critical element of basic mentalizing. Likewise, the appearance or behavior of our pupils can offer revelations about our mental states, as pupil dilation and contraction are entirely involuntary. For instance, our pupils dilate when we show interest. Pupil dilation, particularly in combination with blinking, can be a telltale sign of flirtation. Looking at something or someone we find "attractive" can lower our rate of blinking. Oculesics is influenced by cultural factors. In some cultures, direct eye contact is seen as a sign of anger or disrespect, while in other countries avoiding eye contact is seen as a sign of shame or dishonesty.

"**Vocalics**," a form of paralanguage or prosody, refers to a component of speech beyond the spoken words that modifies meaning, provide nuanced meaning, or convey emotion. Vocalics can be used to clarify, strengthen, or soften messages. The term vocalics pertains to the auditory manner in which something is said, which offers clues to how the message should be interpreted. For instance, a raised voice, staccato vocal pattern, or sarcastic tone may add a layer of meaning which is neither pure body language nor spoken language. Vocalics actually provide the most reliable nonverbal clues with regard to lie detection.

"**Haptics**" pertains to the use and understanding of touch as a communication system. As noted by Sachs (1988) "[t]ouch is the foundation for communication with the world around us, and probably the single sense that is as old as life itself." We can infer mental states in others by observing their self-touch behavior. For instance, when people are afraid, they might put their hand on their throat, and when they feel fatigued, they might rub their forehead. Interpersonal touch can display information about the way we relate to one another. Heslin (1974) categorizes touch into five distinct types. Ranging from impersonal to intimate, they are:

1. Functional/professional touch (e.g., medical examination, physiotherapy)
2. Social/polite touch (e.g., handshake)
3. Friendship/warmth touch (e.g., hug)
4. Love/intimacy touch (e.g., non-sexual kiss or caress)
5. Sexual/arousal touch (e.g., sexual kissing and caressing, intercourse)

Touch can be used to imply dominance, or to offer consolation. Handshakes are a well-known subcategory of haptics. In many cultures, handshakes are common ritualistic touches displayed when people greet each other or when they say goodbye. They also serve to signify transition from one stage to another. For instance, we often shake hands to congratulate people on their success, or to conclude negotiations that result in an agreement. People tend to have their own handshake styles. Touch can also communicate mental states such as trust, affect and confidence.

"**Proxemics**" and "**territoriality**" relate to the use of space and distance as a means of communication, and specifically as an instrument to communicate ownership or occupancy of areas and possessions. Edward T. Hall, a well-known cultural anthropologist who coined the term "proxemics" in 1963, described the interpersonal distances of human beings as falling into four distinct zones. From most intimate to most distant, they are:

1. Intimate space, for embracing, touching, or whispering
2. Personal space, for interactions among good friends or family
3. Social space, for interactions among acquaintances
4. Public space, used for public speaking

Hall also proposed the proximity ranges of these zones, which may vary depending on cultural background. People who live in high contact cultures, such as Latin America and the Mediterranean, tend to express themselves through physical touch, whereas people who live in low contact cultures, such as Asia and Northern Europe, tend to eschew physical contact in favor of maintaining and respecting personal space. The social distance between people correlates significantly with physical distance, and therefore the physical spacing that people maintain can provide social information about their relationships. Haptics and proxemics (including territoriality) are two closely related codes. Together, haptics and proxemics form the "contact codes." They reveal where people reside on the approach-avoidance continuum. This relationship is important for mentalization, as approach and avoidance behaviors indicate the intention to affiliate and cooperate, or to dissociate and/or compete.

"**Chronemics**" - our use of time - is a crucial, yet often overlooked, variable of nonverbal behavior. Psychological time orientation relates to our ideas and expectations about time. It varies from person to person, and from culture to culture. Sometimes we use time as a signal of status. For instance, a person of higher status will make a person of lower status wait for an appointment or a reply.

Our identities and our level of psychological, physical and social well-being are expressed through "**physical appearance**," "**olfactics**," (smells) and "**objectics**." These are all behaviors that intentionally or unintentionally make an impression on others. Although most people associate olfactics with, for instance, perfumes or colognes, we also seem to "read" a person on a much more subconscious level. Research at the Weizmann Institute (Frumin et al., 2015) has revealed that handshakes should be categorized not only under haptics, but also under olfactics because they serve, concomitantly, as a means of transferring "social chemical signals" between people. It appears that people have a tendency to smell their own hand after shaking hands with someone else. Further, we use "objectics," which pertain to object language, the communicative use of material objects (e.g., adornments, the furniture that we use to decorate our house, or the artwork that we display). These representative expressions of identity help to reinforce our identities even more. For instance, we shape our surroundings to express our identity, and our surroundings, in turn, shape our experiences and behavior. While we may overlook these "identity indicators," they can, nevertheless, be very revealing, as they tend to reflect our physiological, psychological and sociological disposition. The mental states we experience in reaction to those identity indicators also reveal information about ourselves, for instance, our attitude toward the identity markers that others display or our own sense of identity in comparison to them.

Another area of nonverbal behavior related to the expression of our identity is "**biological motion**." Researchers on biological motion focus their attention on our perception of motion. One way they do this is by filming individuals who have "point sources" of light attached to their limbs, and examining their movement frame by frame. As explained by Cutting (2013, p. 12), these studies revealed that "we all have a personal signature in our movements." We can guess someone's cultural background or gender by looking at body motion exclusively. Likewise, people can guess who is approaching just by listening to the sound of their gait. Body movements, therefore, play an important role in identity perception.

"**Physiological responses**" in the form of breathing, swallowing, blushing, blanching and sweating – are useful indicators to gauge a person's level of tension. Tension indicators are regularly mentioned as reliable sources to gauge a person's honesty, and although these physiological displays can be exhibited during dishonest or deceitful behavior, most of the time they merely indicate tension. Moreover, signs of tension can result from the stress of being wrongly accused. Blushing is, in general, related to shyness or embarrassment, while blanching is associated with fear. When it comes to breathing, generally speaking, slow, deep breathing indicates a relaxed and confident state of mind, while rapid, shallow breathing indicates an anxious or nervous state of mind. Mimicking the breathing pattern of another person can make us feel similar to the other person, and therefore can be used as a way to connect and resonate with others. We can, in turn, infect others with our breathing pattern, as this behavior tends to be readily shared and embodied by others. We can display a slower, deeper breathing pattern as a means of calming others around us during stressful situations. This is a clear example of affective contagion.

All of the information transmitters that we have discussed help us to piece together critical details that we need for social understanding and interaction. We have divided these critical details, which we refer to as nonverbal social indicators, into three categories:

1. General social indicators
2. Affect indicators
3. Intent indicators

We will now relate the manner in which these three categories of nonverbal social indicators factor into basic mentalizing.

General Social Indicators

"General social indicators" are "general" in that they are *stable* throughout our interactions with others. General social indicators guide our behavior so that we act in a socially acceptable way. Moreover, these nonverbal indicators influence our first impressions of others and the impressions we want to make on others. They help us to understand how to introduce ourselves and how to initiate interactions with others considering the behavioral rules that apply in the particular context. Additionally, they help us to gauge our social bonds with others and the social bonds between other people. In gathering and processing general social indicators, we try to answer the following questions:

First, *with whom am I dealing, and how do I compare with those around me*? The gathering of these social indicators helps us to form a "first impression" of others. A clothing style, for instance, often reveals a certain profession or social standing, and behavioral rituals can help us to infer affiliation with a certain belief system. These indicators also give us insight into how others might judge us in comparison to themselves.

Second, *how do I relate to others, how do others relate to me and how do others relate to each other*? In asking these questions, we are trying to ascertain "social ties." By social ties, we mean connections among people that guide their sharing of experiences, resources and information. These ties can be weak, strong, or latent, depending on the extent and nature of exchanges and interactions between people. To illustrate, using relationship indicators we try to infer the status of others, we attempt to gauge the "dominance/submission balance" between two people or within a group. We also try to estimate the strength of relationships and to determine the kind of exchanges, such as love, resources, information, etc., upon which the relationships are based. Predictions and explanations of behavior should not be made without taking social ties, or the social network of people, into account. Wellman (1988) even went so far as to assert that intrapersonal characteristics of people are *less* important than interpersonal relationships when predicting behavior, as the social network presents opportunities for, and imposes constraints on, people and their behavior. If two people behave similarly, it suggests that their social networks are similar.

Third, *what is expected of me, what can I expect of others and how do I behave appropriately*? Here, we look for social indicators that help us to understand the norms, expectations and standards of the society in which we operate. We also try to detect indicators that reveal a culture's behavioral and emotional display rules, communication customs and etiquettes. We do this particularly to avoid social faux pas. The facial expressions, body movements and body postures of others that reveal a mental state of approval or disapproval help us to understand whether or not we are behaving appropriately. People indicate approval or disapproval of behavior through nonverbal expressions that indicate confusion, disbelief, interest, impatience, irritation, etc.

Affect Indicators

The second category of nonverbal social indicators includes nonverbal "affect indicators," which reveal the emotions, feelings and moods of people. These indicators help us to understand the affective mental states of others, and they help us to become aware of their influence on our own mental states and behavior. Affect indicators also supply social information that influences the formation of epistemic mental states such as desires, beliefs and knowledge, and more complex mental states such as intentions, motivations and attitudes. Affect signals and cues shape our behavior by showing us what is appreciated and what is unwelcome.

Often, we look to facial expressions and body posture/movement to infer the affective states of others. Vocal tone, rhythm, pace and intensity, however, are also very reliable indicators that can be used to gauge the affective states of others. Visceral affect codes such as breathing patterns, swallowing, blushing, blanching and sweating help us to assess a person's level of comfort or discomfort. In gathering affect indicators, we try to answer the following questions:

First, *what is the affective state of the other person*? This question is particularly relevant when the affective state of the other could influence our own affective state, or when our objectives could be impacted by the affective state of the other person. For example, when we need the cooperation or approval of others, we would be wise to approach them at a time they are in an agreeable mood.

Second, *is the other person attempting to bring about a particular change in my behavior through the displayed affect*? Affective displays are powerful communication tools that we can use to shape the behavior of others.

Third, *how is the other person experiencing a situation or interaction*? Understanding how someone experiences something helps us to infer the mental states and explain the behavior of that person. Decoding these affect indicators can reveal the impact people have on one another. This, in turn, functions as an "advance warning system," alerting us to the fact that our interactions are becoming emotionally charged and our mentalization faculties might be taken offline.

Fourth, *is the other person relaxed, or are there signs of distress*? Signs of nervousness, distress, or discomfort in another person can be indicative of an internal conflict, cognitive dissonance, or worrisome mind. Signs of distress can indicate that we need to dig a little deeper. They can also be indicators of physical distress. Moreover, indicators of nervousness might reveal information about someone's dishonest intent.

Fifth, *is the other person showing their true affective state*? In general, we adhere to "emotional display rules" that tell us when to express, suppress, exaggerate, or conceal our emotions. In certain critical cases, however, it is crucial to discern the difference between a sincere emotional display and one that is feigned. In order to make this assessment, we need to look for "emotional leakage," which is most easily recognized in nonverbal signals. This is especially true for hard-to-control emotional "micro expressions," first described by Paul Ekman, a pioneer in the study of emotions and their relation to facial expressions. Ekman and Friesen (1969) identified "facial expressions that occur within a fraction of a second." They further posited that "[t]his involuntary emotional leakage exposes a person's true emotions." For instance, people manage their own affect and emotional expressions, for purposes of presenting themselves in a particular light, or in order to meet contextual demands. To illustrate, it is possible to detect whether someone is genuinely smiling or is faking a smile by looking at the contraction muscles that raise the corners of the mouth and the cheeks, and that form "crow's feet" around the eyes. This is known as a "Duchenne smile." The Duchenne smile has been associated with positive feelings. Studies have shown, however, that a Duchenne smile can be faked, although an exaggerated Duchenne smile is associated with lying. When nonverbal language does not match a person's verbal account, or seems to be out of place in light of the situation or context, either something is amiss, or our expectations of how someone should react are inaccurate. In either instance, further inquiry is warranted. In particular, when we are dealing with people whose cultural background differs significantly from our own, we often misinterpret their nonverbal behavior as being incongruent with their verbal accounts, or with the situation. These misconceptions can have deleterious consequences when we need to judge the trustworthiness of others.

Intent Indicators

The third category of nonverbal social indicators, "intent indicators," is comprised of signals and cues from which we can infer someone's intentions. Intent indicator detection involves the ability to discern whether the behavior of another person has any underlying intention (goal), or whether it was exhibited in an arbitrary manner with no particular goal in mind. Moreover, we need to accurately infer what the intentions of others are in order to predict or explain their behavior. Basic mentalizing, as the name suggests, is focused on the detection of the more basic intent indicators that are conveyed nonverbally. At the basic mentalizing level, we pay particular attention to "*present*-directed intentions," as revealed by actions or behavior that are aimed at the attainment of an immediate goal, as opposed to "*future*-directed intentions" (prior intentions) that are usually detached from the present situation or action. In gathering "intent indicators," we try to answer the following questions:

First, *what does this person need or want*? Through their intentional behavior, strengthened by their affective behavioral expressions, people often try to influence the behavior of others that will assist the influencer in achieving a goal. For example, when people feel that others are not treating them with respect, they might alter their nonverbal behavior in an attempt to elicit more respect from others. We also use intentional indicators to determine whether we can, or even want to, work together with someone.

This brings us to a related line of inquiry: *Is the other person motivated to affiliate or cooperate with me*? Alternatively, *is the other person trying to move away from me, or compete against me*? To answer these questions, we look for indicators that reveal relational messages from which we infer aspects such as intimacy and affection, or dominance and power. We look for signs that indicate whether someone wants to associate with us, or dissociate from us. These signals tell us what people are looking for in others, what they want to share with others, or what they want to avoid. They also predict whether someone is inclined to empathize with us and show compassion if we are in need.

The third line of inquiry: *Can we trust this person; and is this person competent and morally sound*? We look for signs that indicate whether someone will, and is able to, follow through on their commitments, whether they are misrepresenting their identity (pretending to be someone who they are not), whether they are otherwise honest and trustworthy, and whether they have the intention to treat us well and do us no harm.

DETECTING RELEVANT INDICATORS IS NOT EASY

We need to keep in mind that detecting and decoding relevant nonverbal social indicators as a means of mental state reasoning is not easy or straightforward. Almost all of the involuntary indicators, such as pupil dilation, are very difficult to detect. Also, various signals and cues can be susceptible to different interpretations. Further complicating the task, human beings are very much inclined to assign meaning to *arbitrary* cues exhibited by others. Sometimes, however, a yawn is just a yawn, not an intentional signal of boredom or disinterest. The detection and decoding of relevant nonverbal behavior within different socioeconomic layers of society, or across different cultures, has proven to be especially challenging. Even the basic human emotions (e.g., happiness, surprise, anger, fear) are found to be expressed differently in distinct cultural settings, even to the extent that they can be easily misinterpreted by an outsider (see Crivelli et al., 2016). The less elementary the behavior, the more subject to cultural norms and regulations the behavior will be, in terms of its expressions, making accurate interpretation increasingly difficult. Thus, our competency in detecting and decoding nonverbal behavior often requires retooling when we encounter new people with whom we have not yet developed a behavioral baseline. We need to remain mindful of the fact that when we meet people for the first time, we tend to base our judgments about them on heuristics. This does not necessarily present a problem as long as we test our heuristics against all of the available social indicators in order to reduce the likelihood of mistaken impressions based on prejudice, stereotypes and bias.

Now that we have provided an overview of the importance of detecting nonverbal social indicators for basic mentalizing, we will continue with a description of the key advantages, impediments and avenues for enhancement of this ability.

Nonverbal Social Indicator Detection Skills: Advantages, Impediments and Avenues for Enhancement

ADVANTAGES

On an intrapersonal level, *an increased awareness of nonverbal social indicators provides us with a clear view of our own nonverbal displays.* Our self-monitoring level increases, fostering a sense of control over our own nonverbal behavior. Possessing the understanding and capacity to regulate our own nonverbal behavior affects everything, from our ability to make ourselves understood, to the quality of our social life and relationships, to our power to influence the mental states and behavior of others.

On an interpersonal level, *more effective use of information revealed through nonverbal social indicators enhances our interactions with other people.* We consider how our own nonverbal behavior affects others and vice versa. We are better equipped to create positive impressions of warmth, dependability and supportiveness, all aspects associated with social and professional maturity. We are also better able to judge the social competence and trustworthiness of other people. Moreover, we are better equipped to accurately interpret the intentions of others. We make more informed affiliation decisions - whom to befriend, or whom to avoid. We detect signs that suggest a willingness to cooperate, an intention to compete, or a dishonest intent.

On an extrapersonal level, *the ability to encode and decode nonverbal social signals is critical to influencing or understanding larger groups of people,* for example, when giving a speech, creating a corporate image, or conducting observational research in the field of psychology or sociology. Applying these encoding and decoding skills, cultural differences in nonverbal behavior become more recognizable and we are better equipped to identify how these differences impact intercultural social interaction. Finally, we can more readily adjust our nonverbal behavior to fit situational and contextual demands, thereby avoiding social faux pas.

IMPEDIMENTS

There are, however, a number of impediments to encoding, and to detecting and decoding, social nonverbal behavior. From an intrapersonal perspective, research indicates that, generally speaking, *the average person does not pay sufficient attention to nonverbal behavior*. Moreover, *we often fail to detect "negative signals,"* i.e., nonverbal behavior that is conspicuous by its *absence*, such as the absence of a reaction to surprising news. It is our natural tendency to fixate on positive information, to notice what we can sense, as opposed to noticing what is missing. We also tend to direct our attention to nonverbal channels that are easy to detect, for instance facial expressions, leaving a wealth of additional information, such as object language, untapped. Additionally, *our psychophysiological makeup*, e.g., gender, physical limitations, personality traits, intelligence level, etc., *can influence our ability to encode and decode nonverbal behavior*. By way of illustration, studies reveal that the proficiency of a person's *decoding* skills can vary with mental ability and age. Interestingly, research has indicated that *encoding* skills are *unrelated* to race, education, or intelligence.

From an interpersonal perspective, *human beings are predisposed to interpret unintentional nonverbal behavior as intentional*. A further challenge stems from the fact that social signals and cues differ considerably in their encoding and decoding potential. *Some indicators*, such as pupil dilation, *are not as easy and straightforward* to use or make sense of, as are facial expressions or tone of voice. It is particularly difficult to decode social signals that are easily masked, minimized, exaggerated, or substituted. We need to keep in mind that, although many nonverbal signals or patterns of behavior have commonly accepted interpretations, these meanings may nevertheless require *clarification* or *verification* between sender and receiver.

From an extrapersonal perspective, people who work or live in a multicultural environment will likely encounter these challenges on a more frequent basis, as *nonverbal behavior can have a different meaning from one culture to another*. Additionally, *context may diminish our opportunity to encode and decode signals and cues*. For instance, the use of virtual meeting technologies may prevent people from seeing or hearing each other well enough to make effective use of the full range of nonverbal social indicators.

AVENUES FOR ENHANCEMENT

Individuals vary substantially in their nonverbal encoding and decoding abilities. Research tells us that encoding and decoding skills are correlated to a certain extent. Better encoders tend to be better decoders, and vice versa. Therefore, gains in one area can translate into improvement in the other. *Maturation, experience, training* and *instruction* improve our ability to encode and decode nonverbal behavior. Let us look at how we can enhance these abilities.

There are four main vectors along which we can hone our nonverbal encoding and decoding competencies. The first vector involves *the objective assessment of our nonverbal behavior decoding and encoding competencies.* With regard to our decoding of nonverbal behavior, we need to gain an accurate perspective of how well we detect relevant social signals and cues of others so that we can accurately mentalize about them. In relation to encoding our nonverbal behavior, insight into the clarity and effectiveness of our nonverbal behavior is equally essential as it helps other people accurately mentalize about us.

The second vector is aimed at *improving our own ability to detect and decode the nonverbal behavior of others.* Nonverbal social signals and cues provide a rich source of input to the mentalization process. But these valuable clues are wasted if we are oblivious to them. Once again, we need to keep in mind that nonverbal indicators can come in many different forms, as people have at their disposal a variety of nonverbal encoding channels. We also need to be on the lookout for nonverbal behavior that is *inconsistent* with the situation or context, including *omitted* behavior that we would expect to see under the circumstances. In terms of decoding, we need to recognize that nonverbal signals and cues can be susceptible to more than one interpretation. Factors such as cultural and socioeconomic background can have a strong influence on both the nonverbal behavior itself and the interpretation of that behavior. It is important to remember that we do not decode signals and cues in a vacuum. What we glean from one sensory channel needs to be validated against input that we receive from our other senses. This enables us to gain a more holistic picture of what others are trying to communicate. Our capacity for attentional control and flexibility enables us to focus on the behavior of others, while at the same time, monitoring additional situational factors, such as our own behavior and mental states and circumstantial influences.

The third vector focuses on *sharpening our nonverbal encoding and delivery skills*. We have to be aware of the full range of nonverbal communication channels through which we convey social information. We need to use these channels appropriately to convey our own nonverbal messages clearly and effectively. For instance, it is important to create the right ambiance for a healthy exchange of nonverbal social signals and cues. When we create the right "sharing" environment, meaningful nonverbal behavior (as is the case with verbal behavior) often flows freely from others. We can do this through our own displays of positive nonverbal behavior. People find positive nonverbal behavior to be *appealing* and *inviting*. Displays of positive nonverbal behavior create an environment of comfort, dignity and receptiveness. By displaying such behavior, we will be viewed as approachable and receptive. "Defensive body language," on the other hand, discourages people from engaging with us. When our nonverbal behavior suggests a sense of disinterest towards others, we will most likely be perceived by others as unapproachable or, worse yet, rude. Nor do we want to come across as authoritarian, as such an impression tends to stifle the sharing of personal information by others.

References

American Psychological Association. (n.d.). Barnum-effect. In *APA dictionary of psychology*. Retrieved July 17, 2022, from https://dictionary.apa.org/barnum-effect

Birdwhistell, R. L. (1952), *Introduction to kinesics: An annotated system for the analysis of body motion and gesture*. Louisville, KY: University of Louisville.

Crivelli, C., Jarillo, S., Russell, J. A., & Fernández-Dols, J. M. (2016). Reading emotions from faces in two indigenous societies. *Journal of Experimental Psychology: General, 145*(7), 830–843. doi:10.1037/xge0000172

Cutting, J. E. (2013). *People Watching: Social, Perceptual, and Neurophysiological Studies of Body Perception* (Johnson, K. L. & Shiffrar, M. (Ed.). Oxford University Press.

Ekman, P., & Friesen, W. V. (1969). "Nonverbal Leakage and Clues to Deception". *Journal for the Study of Interpersonal Processes, 32*(1): 88–106. doi:10.1080/00332747.1969.11023575

Frumin, I., Ofer Perl, O., Endevelt-Shapira, Y., Eisen, A., Eshel, N., Heller, I., Shemesh, M., Ravia, A., Sela, L., Arzi, A., & Sobel, N. (2015). A Social Chemosignaling Function for Human Handshaking. *eLife Sciences*, 3(4): e05154. doi: 10.7554/eLife.05154.

Hall, E. T. (1963a). "Proxemics-the study of man's spatial relations," in *Man's image in medicine and anthropology*. Edited by I. Galdston, pp. 422-45. New York: International Universities Press.

Heslin, R. (1974, May). *Steps toward a taxomony of touching.* Paper presented to the annual meeting of the Midwestern Psychological Association, Chicago, IL.

Sachs, F. (1988). The intimate sense. *Sciences, 28*(1), 28-34. doi:10.1002/J.2326-1951.1988.TB02993.X

Wellman, B., & Berkowitz, S. D. (Eds.). (1988). *Structural analysis in the social sciences, Vol. 2. Social structures: A network approach*. Cambridge University Press.

SECTION II.

BASIC MENTALIZING

To Sense and Perceive

Chapter 3.

Nonsocial Sensing and Associating

Alexithymia

Fluctuations in nonsocial sensing are often observed during the most severe manifestations of psychological dysfunctions, for instance, during a major depression. Altered interoception might be related to a disorder in the ability to perceive and express emotions, as is the case with "alexithymia" or "hypochondriasis," two conditions where people exhibit defects in perceiving and describing their own affective or physical states.

Let us take a closer look at alexithymia. Nemiah (1977) describes "alexithymia" as a subclinical phenomenon involving difficulty in identifying, processing, describing and dealing with one's own feelings or the feelings of others. It is accompanied by difficulty in distinguishing between *feelings* and *bodily sensations* of arousal. Alexithymia literally means "no words for feelings." It is, however, a multifaceted construct that encompasses more difficulties than simply the inability to find appropriate words to describe feelings. Sifneos (1973) mentions the following key features related to this disorder: "a relative constriction in emotional functioning, poverty of fantasy life, and inability to find appropriate words to describe their emotions." When a person is described as a "human robot," or an "emotional illiterate," it might be that this individual is suffering from alexithymia. It is an uncommon disorder that can significantly impact many aspects of a person's life. People suffering from alexithymia feel something, but they are unable to distinguish in any real way what that feeling is. Because the associations do not come naturally, most of their emotional displays are learned responses. People who suffer from alexithymia may put on a smile during a happy event, such as a wedding, because they know they are expected to behave that way, even though it does not feel natural to them. There are two distinct subtypes of alexithymia, *primary alexithymia,* which refers to "a life-long dispositional factor that can lead to psychosomatic illness" (Lesser, 1981), and *secondary alexithymia* resulting from developmental arrests due to sociocultural conditioning or as a coping mechanism by cause of "massive psychological trauma in childhood or later on in life" (Taylor et al., 1997). Individuals diagnosed with secondary alexithymia are more likely to respond to therapy or training than individuals who suffer from primary alexithymia. This disorder is associated with deficits in both *empathy* and *theory of mind,* and therefore has a negative impact on all three mentalization levels.

The challenges presented by alexithymia demonstrate the importance of accurate interoceptive and exteroceptive association in connection with mentalization.

As you know by now, basic mentalizing is our most elementary level of mentalization. Basic mentalizing relies upon stimuli coming from both inside and outside of our body. These nonverbal signals and cues are generally processed without conscious awareness. They provide us with discernible information from which we can infer mental states. In the previous chapters, we discussed the embodied sharing of affect and behavior, and the detection of nonverbal social indicators. In this third and final chapter of basic mentalizing, we explain the sensing and associating of nonsocial interoceptive and exteroceptive stimuli. Interoceptive and exteroceptive sensing and associating is discussed in this chapter in relation to "nonsocial" signals and cues in the sense that they do not require social interaction. Nevertheless, they can influence the way we perceive ourselves, others and situations, as they are strongly embodied.

Nonsocial Interoceptive and Exteroceptive Awareness

Humans have a wide variety of sensory channels that help them to make sense of the world around them, and their inner world. "Nonsocial sensing" pertains to our ability to detect stimuli *outside* of social interaction that come from within and outside of our body, respectively referred to as interoceptive and exteroceptive awareness. Let us start by examining interoceptive awareness. The perception of stimuli coming from within the body is known as "interoception." "**Interoceptive awareness**" of visceral and bodily changes can be seen as a type of "paying attention." Interoception includes not only visceral sensations, but also all sensory signals that convey information about the state of the body, including the skin, the musculoskeletal system and hormonal state. "Visceral factors" are states of being, such as hunger, thirst, physical pain and various arousals that are connected to an affective state. Interoceptive information is important to answer the question "*How do I feel*?" It influences how and how much an interaction, event, or belonging is valued. In a figurative sense, something "visceral" is felt "deep down." It is a "gut feeling," or "intuition." Interoception constitutes an important component of self-representation and emotional experience, as it provides the basis for how we feel and express our emotions. The underlying purpose of interoceptive information is to achieve both "homeostasis," an optimal internal balance, and "allostasis," which involves the dynamic adjustment of homeostasis to ever-changing environments. Interoceptive sensations, including the anticipation of those sensations, prompt us to action. We all have our own "interoceptive signature." For instance, everyone has a distinct heart rate variable, a measure of the *variation* in the beat-to-beat interval. Research studies suggest that a *higher* heart rate variable is associated with better affect regulation and well-being, while a *lower* heart rate variable is associated with worry and anxiety (Kemp & Quintana, 2013).

The perception of stimuli coming from outside of the body is known as "exteroception." "**Exteroceptive awareness**," another type of "paying attention," is focused on external stimuli. Exteroceptive somatosensory perception refers to experiences attributed to external stimuli that come in contact with the body, such as noise, sun rays, atmospheric pressure, wind, texture of clothing, etc. Exteroceptive information is typically conveyed by the skin, the musculoskeletal system and other subsystems - sight, taste, smell, hearing, etc. These external sensory stimuli do *not directly* elicit emotional responses. Their emotional impact is solely dependent on our interpretation of the effect they have on us. As with interoceptive information, exteroceptive information influences the way we think, feel and act. Exteroceptive information connects us to our environment. The capacity for exteroceptive sensing plays a critical role in our tendency to synchronize behavior and affect with others.

Intero- and exteroception enable us to learn about our physical condition and our external surroundings. The sensations that we experience become integrated into our emotions, thoughts and behavioral patterns. These sensations are coined as "somatic markers" by Antonio Damasio (see Damasio et al., 1991), a Portuguese-American neuroscientist who has shown that emotions play a central role in social cognition. For instance, people readily associate the sensation of a rapid heartbeat with anxiety, nausea with disgust, etc. Additionally, somatic markers strongly influence consequent decision-making and strengthen our intuition. Although these physical sensations can have a powerful influence on mental states and behavior, people often fail to recognize their influence. In other words, they do not *anticipate, appreciate,* or even *remember* the influence that these somatic factors have had, or are likely to have, on their perceptions, affect, or behavior.

While intero- and exteroception do help us to make sense of our physical condition and the world around us, they can also bias our perceptions. When we experience interoceptive sensorial states such as hunger and fatigue, or exteroceptive sensorial states such as sensorial overload due to environmental stimuli, otherwise known as being in a "hot state," we tend to focus our attention on goals that are associated with our hot sensorial state, relegating other goals to a secondary status. When we return to a "cold state" - meaning we are no longer under the influence of interoceptive or exteroceptive sensations, we may have a hard time rationalizing our prior behavior. Likewise, if we are in a cold state, we may have a hard time predicting how we will behave if we later find ourselves subject to interoceptive or exteroceptive influences. The same holds true for our interpretation or prediction of the behavior of others. The human tendency we have to underestimate the influences of sensorial drives on the behaviors, attitudes and preferences of ourselves and others is a cognitive bias referred to as the "hot-cold empathy gap." Let us discuss the important components that provide internal feedback about our well-being and about our reactions to external sensory input.

Important Components of Nonsocial Sensing

On the interoceptive side, we start with the "**visceral system**" - the autonomic nervous system that acts largely unconsciously and regulates bodily functions. Important components of the visceral system are:

- The "**cardiovascular system**," an organ system that permits blood to circulate and transports oxygen, carbon dioxide and nutrients. Throughout the body the cardiovascular system also helps in fighting disease and stabilizing temperature. It is measured in terms of heart rate and blood pressure.
- The "**respiratory system**," which consists of specific organs and structures used for the exchange of oxygen and carbon dioxide. It is measured by breathing pattern and rate.
- The "**gastrointestinal system**," an organ system which takes in food, provides for digestion and expels waste. It provides interoceptive sensations such as hunger, thirst, nausea, etc.
- The "**genito-urinary system**," the organ system consisting of the reproductive organs and the urinary system.
- The "**endocrine**" and "**immune systems**," which detect, interpret and respond to threats to the body, and regulate homeostasis. The endocrine system helps us identify our level of arousal or stress.

Basic mentalizing efforts focus on nonverbal behavior to detect physical changes that are indicative of stress levels. Furthermore, we interpret the emotions we feel on the basis of our visceral responses to situational aspects.

Additionally, there are components of the interoceptive sensory system that overlap with components of our exteroceptive sensory system, such as:

- The "**thermoregulatory system**," which maintains body temperature within certain boundaries, notwithstanding fluctuations in the surrounding environment. Signs of the thermoregulatory system at work include sweating, shivering and blushing.

- The "**chemoreceptive system**," which converts chemical substances in the internal or external environment of the human body into biological signals. It allows us, for instance, to detect signs of fear or anxiousness through our sense of smell.
- The "**nociceptive system**," which allows for the receiving and processing of pain-inducing stimuli originating either within or outside of the body. Interestingly, psychological pain induced by social rejection is processed in the same brain regions that process physical pain. In that sense, social rejection is similar to physical injury.
- "**Proprioception**," or body awareness, which relies upon sensory input from muscles and joints through muscle contractions and movement. It provides information about where a certain body part is, and how it is moving and oriented in relation to the environment.
- The "**vestibular system**," which consists of a collection of components situated in the inner ear, and provides feedback related to body motion and spatial orientation.
- The "**integumentary system**," the body's outer layer consisting of skin, hair, nails and glands, which provides both valuable interoceptive and exteroceptive information. In relation to interoception, sensations from this system can indicate your state of well-being, as illustrated by your skin sensitivity when you come down with the flu. It also provides intuitive information of how we feel about others or situations (e.g., the feeling you get when someone or something makes your skin crawl or your hair stand on end, or gives you goosebumps). The integumentary system is also critical when it comes to touch, an exteroceptive sensing element described next.

Finally, there are components that predominantly belong to the exteroceptive sensory systems. The exteroceptive sensorial systems pertain to the senses that gather information from the external world. They help us to create a perception of the world around us. These components consist of:

- The "**tactile system**" - our sense of touch, which provides qualitative information (texture, temperature, pressure, vibration) about people and objects we come in close contact with.
- The "**gustatory system**" - our sense of taste, which provides information about different aspects of flavor (whether something tastes sweet, salty, bitter, etc.).
- The "**olfactory system**" - our sense of smell, which provides information about different aspects of odors (whether something smells musty, acrid, flowery, etc.).
- The "**visual system**" - our sense of sight, which helps us identify objects and detect colors, shapes and motion.
- The "**auditory system**" - our sense of hearing, which provides information about sounds in the environment (whether a noise sounds loud, soft, near, distant, etc.).

Beyond the information provided through conventional sensorial systems, we also gather information through a number of more subjective sensations. "**Intuition**," often referred to as our "gut feeling" or "sixth sense," is a type of knowledge that we develop over the course of our lives. It helps us to make quick decisions without resort to deliberation or more complex reasoning. When we use intuition, it feels as though we knew in advance how a situation was going to unfold, and instantly understood how to respond to that situation. Intuition is different from instinct, as instinct is an innate biological force that impels us to behave in a certain way. By contrast, the intuitive process is learned.

The "**sense of agency**" is derived from the combination of self-awareness and appreciation of one's control over, and responsibility for, behavior and outcomes. The sense of agency supports theory of mind capacities through the self-other distinction that we need to make when mentalizing. It is described by Gallagher (2000) as "the experience that I am the one who is causing or generating the action. For example, the sense that I am the one who is causing something to move, or that I am the one who is generating a certain thought in my stream of consciousness." It is closely integrated with the "**sense of ownership**," described by Gallagher in the same article as "[t]he sense that I am the one who is undergoing an experience. For example, the sense that my body is moving regardless of whether the movement is voluntary or involuntary." Gallagher proposed in his 2000 article that "[p]henomena such as delusions of control, auditory hallucinations, and thought insertion appear to involve problems with the sense of agency rather than the sense of ownership."

The "**sense of familiarity**," is the feeling that a particular person, event, or place is familiar in some way. A strong sense of familiarity can occur without any past exposure, as is the case with déjà vu. The experience of familiarity may itself be a form of intuition. The sense of familiarity may bias our perceptions of others, leading us to falsely attribute qualities to a person on the basis of our perceived foreknowledge of them. We might not make the same effort to truly get to know such a person, and understand their perspectives, as we would, generally speaking, with new acquaintances. We tend to more readily accept things that seem familiar to us than things that are new. The same holds true when it comes to people.

Another often overlooked subjective sensation is the "**sense of time**," the subjective perception of event duration and the passage of time. Time perception is subject to influences of emotional state, level of attention, memory and disease. In general, we all experience these sensations, though most often, they go unnoticed. It is important to become more conscious of our full range of subjective sensations in relation to mentalization.

Accurately attributing sensorial influences to behavior is another critical aspect of mentalizing about others and ourselves. Let us examine the ability to associate intero- and extroceptive sensations accurately with their cause.

Interoceptive and Exteroceptive Information Association

Detecting interoceptive and exteroceptive information is essential, however, associating it correctly with what is happening is equally critical. For example, when experiencing a visceral response related to physical exertion (i.e., climbing stairs) people sometimes misinterpret their physiological responses as the onset of a panic attack, which in turn leads to an intensification of the physiological responses, further increasing feelings of anxiety. The same sort of chain reaction can take place when we "inherit" feelings of anxiety from those around us, but view ourselves as the source of the visceral reaction, a form of affective contagion, as previously discussed.

Just as with interoceptive awareness, exteroceptive informational cues are often mistakenly associated with causes related to the way we, and others, think, feel and act. For instance, sometimes we can feel irritated by the brightness or warmth of the sun without being consciously aware of the source of our irritation. This lack of awareness can lead us to attribute our irritation to the behavior of others, causing us to react in a negative way toward them. Alternatively, we might associate positive environmental stimuli, such as a cool refreshing breeze, with people in our presence, making us more comfortable with them. Thus, faulty associations of this nature can impact our relationships with others, both positively and negatively.

Accurately detecting and associating nonsocial indicators is essential for mentalization. Internal and external nonsocial stimuli influence our decision-making. For instance, when we are fatigued, we are more likely to base our decisions on intuition. Informed by underlying nonsocial sensations, our intuition often guides us toward good decision-making. However, in situations that call for strategic mentalizing, such as complex negotiations, it is better to remain mindful that nonsocial sensations, like fatigue, can actually cloud our decision-making ability. Nonsocial sensations can also decrease our sensitivity to social stimuli. For example, the sensation of pain tends to focus our attention on ourselves rather than on others (unless, of course, the other person is the source of our pain).

In addition to monitoring and regulating our own intero- and exteroceptive sensations, we need to take the intero- and exteroceptive sensations of others into account when we infer their mental states and attempt to explain or predict their behavior. For instance, when we commence a meeting with someone who is already showing signs of stress or irritation, we need to understand that complex or contentious topics may require greater patience and consideration. We also need to determine whether people with whom we interact are aware of their own intero- and exteroceptive sensations, and the influences that those sensations have on their own behavior. Sensory acuity and self-awareness differ significantly from one person to the next. Individuals who are good at detecting and associating nonsocial stimuli are often endowed with a high level of sensory perceptiveness. This is often due to a higher-than-average central nervous system sensitivity, which alerts more readily to nonsocial stimuli, coupled with a capacity for deeper cognitive processing of nonsocial and social signals and cues. This keen sensitivity may be further driven and intensified by a heightened emotional reactivity, both positive and negative. It is not hard to understand how this sensorial keenness can be beneficial for mentalization. However, as with heightened susceptibility to sharing in the affect and behavior of others, sensorial keenness can actually become an impediment to mentalizing if it is not properly channeled and regulated. An overly acute sensory system can cause a person to become overwhelmed, exhausted and inwardly focused, and search for ways to escape the situation.

Impairment in the perception and interpretation of nonsocial sensorial states is associated with a decreased ability to identify and describe one's own emotions and the emotions of others. Moreover, these impairments can cause a person to rely more heavily on laborious deliberative cognitive processes, rather than intuition, to make decisions. This, in turn, can lead such a person to become less exploratory and more rigid, as they tend to find new environments and behaviors far more exhausting than other people do. These difficulties have been associated with disorders like autism and alexithymia. When it comes to the detection and processing of nonsocial stimuli, *achieving the right balance* is critical. Both over- and under-sensitivity can bias our mentalization efforts. *Over*-sensitivity can lead to sensorial overload, which distracts us from effective mentalizing. *Under*-sensitivity can make it harder for us to detect another person's feelings, which inhibits effective mentalizing. More severe sensory processing difficulties or disorders fall under the category of "sensory processing disorders" (SPDs). Though not recognized as an official medical disorder, an SPD undoubtedly affects how our brain processes sensory information.

Sensory processing difficulties manifest themselves in a number of ways. People who are over-sensitive to sensorial input find it difficult to filter out any interoceptive and/or exteroceptive stimuli. As a consequence, they often react poorly to these stimuli. For instance, they may feel overwhelmed or exhausted by the constant stream of sensory data. Such individuals prefer their normal routines over new experiences, and they often need more "alone" time in order to keep their energy levels well balanced. They can display a behavioral disposition that seems lethargic, slow and/or clumsy, giving the impression that they suffer from poor motor skills. These symptoms may undermine such a person's self-confidence and sense of self-efficacy, which in turn can lead to social isolation and even depression. People who are under-sensitive to sensorial input are largely unaware of interoceptive and/or exteroceptive stimuli. These individuals experience a craving for sensory stimulation. They may engage in thrill-seeking behavior (driving at a high speed, scaling heights without a safety rope, etc.). They often display impulsive behavior, fidgeting and/or seeking or making loud, disturbing noises. They tend to overlook social cues, or show a lack of respect for the personal space of others.

One final challenge regarding our sensitivity to sensory data stems from our tendency to assume that other people share our level of sensitivity. The assumption that others experience situations the same way we do can bias the mental state inferences that we draw about others, and influence the accuracy of predictions or explanations we make about their behavior.

Nonsocial Sensing and Associating Acuity: Advantages, Impediments and Avenues for Enhancement

ADVANTAGES

From an intrapersonal perspective, research shows that *the right level of sensorial acuity and awareness enables us to pay the right level of attention and devote the right attentional focus* to the nonsocial data provided by our own senses and experiences. This helps us to recognize those sensations that have the capacity to influence our own mental states and behavior, and understand how these sensations impact our perceptions of others. These are critical aspects of mentalization. Moreover, becoming aware of these dynamics is the first step in honing our ability to control and regulate many of these intero- and exteroceptive sensations.

On an interpersonal level, *the right level of nonsocial sensing acuity helps us to apply well-informed self-other comparisons to account for different sensitivity levels,* another important aspect of mentalization. Similarly, a healthy sensory balance helps us to recognize the sensorial influences that other people are experiencing, and the impact of those influences on their mentalization. In addition, this helps us to treat others, and have others treat us, in a way that suits the sensitivity levels of all parties concerned (for instance, by respecting the need for personal space). In addition, it helps us to close the hot-cold empathy gap, which leads to a better understanding of our own behavior and the behavior of others.

On an extrapersonal level, *having a good understanding of our sensorial makeup helps us to adapt to and shape our environment*. Our sensorial sensitivity provides for essential protective and defensive functions. When we take our sensorial sensitivity into proper account, we are better able to select the right environment to help us thrive. Interculturally, it helps us to understand why people who visit or move to another country might struggle to adjust to factors such as high or low temperatures, densely or sparsely populated environments, or new tastes and smells. We will also be more aware of the challenges presented by virtual meetings with colleagues who work in different time zones. For example, while we might feel relaxed and energetic because our workday has just started, our colleagues in other parts of the world might be tired and ready to go home.

IMPEDIMENTS

A number of impediments can interfere with our sensorial keenness. On an intrapersonal level, *interoceptive stimuli,* such as elevated blood pressure or low blood sugar levels, *are more difficult to detect and control than external stimuli,* such as noise. Likewise, changes in heart rate can be detected more readily than changes in our endocrine system. Another impediment is *sensory overload* or *sensory deprivation* stemming from over- or under-sensitivity. Distracting influences, such as a cluttered or troubled mind, can further impede our sensorial acuity.

Interpersonally, *excessive focus on our own sensorial experience can cause us to lose connection with others.* Likewise, *focusing too much on the sensorial experience of others causes us to lose connection with our own experiential being.* When either connection suffers, we lose our awareness of the impact that our sensorial experiences have on our interaction with others. Detecting the impact of intero- and exteroceptive sensations on others presents an even greater challenge, as they are not, generally speaking, observable without a measuring device.

On an extrapersonal level, impediments can result from *exteroceptive sensations that are so strong and overpowering* (e.g., a very noisy environment or a particularly foul odor) *that all other sensations remain below our awareness threshold.* Additionally, it can be quite difficult to *estimate the intero- and exteroceptive sensations of people who come from cultural backgrounds and experiences that are very different from our own.* We conclude this chapter with an examination of the opportunities that exist for enhancement of our nonsocial sensing and associating abilities.

AVENUES FOR ENHANCEMENT

As previously mentioned, our sensory system serves a protective and defensive function. It keeps us in proper balance and safe from danger. If we become overwhelmed by sensorial stimuli, our central nervous system can initiate a "fight, flight, or freeze" reaction, resulting in physiological responses, such as sweating, increased heart rate, pupil dilation, etc. Overwhelming sensations can take our mentalization faculties offline. Learning how to rebalance our nervous system in the wake of a disruptive sensory experience promotes the restoration of those faculties. Understanding these brain-body interactions is essential to mentalizing for yet another reason. It gives us insight into how we can manage our senses optimally to infer mental states. In addition, it reduces the risk that our sensations will be misread, or that they will bias our perceptions by negatively impacting our emotions, our behavior and our ability to mentalize. Effective information gathering, both social and nonsocial, can be improved by regulating the flow and focus of energy that we allocate to the information gathering process.

Our sensory detection and association processes can be enhanced in a systematic manner. The first step is to *establish a baseline* by assessing our sensitivity to interoceptive and exteroceptive sensations, and our ability to associate these sensations accurately with their internal and external sources. The second step is to *strengthen our attentional focus and orientation.* This involves our ability to direct our attentional focus to the various sensations coming from within and outside of our body. We can improve our sensorial awareness by employing a more volitional, responsive "top down" approach, rather than a reactive "bottom up" approach. The third step is to *enhance our detection abilities.* Here, we focus on detecting the presence or absence of stimuli, such as shallow breathing or numbness. At this point, we must decide whether to attend to or ignore a sensation. By ignoring extraneous sensations, we can concentrate on improving our estimation of the quality, intensity, or duration of more relevant stimuli. This third step, known as "registration," allows us to identify where the intero- or exteroceptive stimuli originate. The fourth step is to *enhance the accuracy of our associations.*

This is the point at which we assign meaning to stimuli. Instinct, intuition, situational memories and present mental states all influence our interpretation and resultant appraisal of the current situation. The accuracy of our detection and association of nonsocial stimuli is closely linked to the fifth step which involves our ability to *respond in the most effective and appropriate way*. Here we decide whether or not a response is required, and how to respond most appropriately. The response can be cognitive, affective, or behavioral, or a blend of all three. The sixth and final step involves *regular self-reflection* on our own sensorial experiences and the impact they have on our mentalizing activities.

Additionally, we need to enhance our awareness of sensory overload or sensory deprivation that others might experience. We also need to learn how to recognize the impact of intero- and exteroceptive stimuli on the perspectives of others and help them to associate their sensorial experiences accurately.

SECTION SUMMARY

As we conclude this final basic mentalizing chapter, we would like to summarize what we have discussed thus far in this section. We have introduced you to the three components of basic mentalizing. In the first chapter, we explained how we can infer mental states from our primitive tendency to share in affect (i.e., the experience of feelings, moods, or emotions), and to synchronize our behavior with people around us. In the second chapter, we examined our ability to infer mental states through social indicators that are conveyed nonverbally - such as gestures, postures and facial expressions - without the requirement for embodied sharing. In this final chapter, we discussed nonsocial sensing and associating involving our interoceptive and exteroceptive sensing systems. Here, we focused on the gathering of information which, while nonsocial, can nevertheless have a considerable impact on our ability to mentalize about ourselves and others, and on the accuracy of our inferences. In the following section, we are going to discuss the next level of mentalization: "affective mentalizing."

References

Damasio, A. R., Tranel, D., & Damasio, H., (1991). Somatic markers and the guidance of behaviour: theory and preliminary testing. In Levin, H. S., Eisenberg, H. M., Benton, A.L. (Eds.), *Frontal Lobe Function and Dysfunction.* Oxford University Press, New York, pp. 217–229.

Gallagher, S. (2000). Philosophical conceptions of the self: implications for cognitive science. *Trends in Cognitive Sciences, 4(1), 14–21.* doi:10.1016/s1364-6613(99)01417-5

Kemp., A. H., & Quintana D. S. (2013). The relationship between mental and physical health: Insights from the study of heart rate variability. *International Journal of Psychophysiology, 89*(3), 288–296. doi: 10.1016/j.ijpsycho.2013.06.01

Lesser, I. M. (1981). A Review of the Alexithymia Concept. *Psychosomatic Medicine, 43*(6), *531–543.* doi:10.1097/00006842-198112000-00009

Nemiah, J. C. (1977). Alexithymia. Theoretical considerations. *Psychother Psychosomatics, 28*(1-4), 199-206. doi: 10.1159/000287064.

Sifneos, P. E. (1973). The Prevalence of 'Alexithymic' Characteristics in Psychosomatic Patients. *Psychotherapy and Psychosomatics,* 22(2-6), 255–262. doi:10.1159/000286529

Taylor, G. J., Bagby, R. M., & Parker, J. D. A. (1997). *Disorders of affect regulation: Alexithymia in medical and psychiatric illness.* Cambridge University Press. https://doi.org/10.1017/CBO9780511526831

SECTION III.

AFFECTIVE MENTALIZING

To Simulate and Project

Chapter 1.

Attitude Toward Affect and Affective Understanding

Introduction to Affective Mentalizing

We begin this chapter by reviewing where affective mentalizing fits within the full scope of mentalization. At the affective mentalizing level, we consciously monitor the affective mental states (feelings, moods and emotions) of ourselves and others. This conscious monitoring allows us to *regulate our own affective states* and to *influence the affective states of others.* Affective mentalizing enables us to focus in on the affective aspects of our interactions with others, and to show empathy and compassion, or invite the same from others, when required. Affective mentalizing is a highly critical competence, as a stressful affective state can trigger a fight, flight, or freeze reaction, impeding our ability and willingness to understand others, and disrupting our mentalization efforts. In addition, affective mentalizing is critical to assuring that our mentalization faculties remain online, even when we are distracted or fatigued.

It is on this mentalization level that we integrate *nonverbal* affect indicators, gathered through basic mentalizing activities, with *verbal* affective information to gain an accurate understanding of what is going on, from an affective perspective, in our own mind and in the minds of others. Affective mentalizing can be further seen as an "immediate antecedent" for strategic mentalizing, the level at which affective information is incorporated into increasingly *rational models* of intention and motivation. Affective mentalizing also serves as a "hub" for gauging whether basic mentalizing is adequate for the particular situation, or whether we need to advance to strategic mentalizing. We are often prompted to migrate from one level of mentalization to another by affective verbal and nonverbal indicators that we detect in ourselves, or in others. For instance, a sense of agitation, confusion and tension often indicate an underlying affective mental state that warrants additional mentalization bandwidth.

Two key features of affective mentalizing are simulation and projection. "**Simulation**" involves embodying the affect of others in order to better understand how they experience a situation. Simulation initially starts below our level of consciousness through mimicry, affective contagion and behavioral contagion, before leading us to empathize with others. "**Projection**," on the other hand, entails a cognitive effort from the outset to understand the affective mental states of others by "projecting" ourselves into the same situation. With projection, we use our own feelings, thoughts and experiences as a proxy for those of others. This is what is meant by *"putting yourself in the shoes of another person,"* an essential prerequisite for empathizing with others. Armed with the "ready-made" affective understanding provided by simulation and projection, we can very effectively manage feelings, moods and emotions. If the situation becomes more complex, however, we need to apply our higher-level strategic mentalizing competencies, which enable us to think more rationally about what is going on in the minds of others. When we find it hard to empathize with others, we might benefit from applying our basic mentalizing competencies, which increase our susceptibility to affective contagion.

Besides simulation and projection, many of the key features of basic and strategic mentalizing are represented in this intermediate level as well, although to a more moderate degree, and with a particular focus on affective mental states. Affective mentalizing is, for instance, *slower* than basic mentalizing and *more effortful*. On the other hand, it is *faster* than strategic mentalizing, though in complex circumstances, *more prone to error*. In summary, affective mentalizing offers the following advantages:

- It helps us to detect and regulate fight, flight, or freeze reactions.
- It keeps our mentalization faculties online.
- It helps us to migrate fluidly between levels of mentalization as the situation requires.
- It helps us to reconnect with others and maintain healthy relationships through empathy, compassion and appropriate affective communication.

Affective mentalizing is focused primarily on *establishing or restoring balanced affective states*. Once affective states are stabilized at a well-balanced level, we can shift our focus from relational goals to more instrumental goals. Affective mentalizing consists of three components. Each component will be examined in a separate chapter. In this first chapter, the *impact of attitude toward affect and affective understanding* will be discussed. We will examine how attitude toward affect is formed and how this attitude influences our affective understanding of ourselves and others. Additionally, we will look at how affective understanding, a deeply and broadly developed comprehension of emotions, feelings and moods, increases our ability for complex affective thinking. In the second chapter we will explore the *progression from affective contagion and affect indicator processing to empathizing with others and applying compassionate behavior*. We will examine the difference between two forms of empathy – "affective empathy" and "cognitive empathy" - and the concept of "empathic distress." Additionally, we will examine compassionate behavior. In the third chapter we will explore affective communication. This encompasses the *exchange of affective information between people,* including the capacity to send and receive affective messages appropriately in social interactions. To set the stage for the current chapter, we will now introduce you to a psychological disorder that is closely related to the development of our attitude toward, and understanding of, affect: "affect phobia."

Affect Phobia

Dealing with negative affects like sadness, anger and anxiety can be difficult. In fact, many of us fear these unpleasant emotions and prefer not to deal with them at all. The term "affect phobia" (from Latin "animi motus," meaning "emotion") refers to a debilitating level of fear of *feeling affects* and *expressing emotions*. This phobia encompasses fear of both *positive* and *negative* affects. Emotions of sadness and anger are common fear triggers, as they are closely related to the fear of losing self-control. Sometimes, experiencing a negative emotion on a frequent basis can make a person fearful that the emotion will resurface. People who suffer from affect phobia may have anxiety attacks when experiencing strong emotions. These individuals try to avoid situations that elicit strong affects. Affect phobic symptoms can include overthinking, rapid heartbeat, nausea, trembling, loss of control and loss of sense of reality.

Research in the field of "attachment theory" helps us to explain fundamental causes for this phobia, as these causes are often rooted in our childhood. As we will explain in more detail later in this chapter, caregivers are role models for dealing with feelings, moods and emotions. During childhood we can learn that emotions, particularly negative ones, are "not OK," if our caregivers do not validate our experience and expression of these feelings. This behavior, which can alienate children from their emotional selves, is often accompanied by the caregiver shaming the child for experiencing and/or expressing the emotion. The caregiver may tell a child to stop whining and to be strong, even in situations where negative feelings are entirely appropriate, such as the loss of a pet or a friend. Similarly, the caregiver may ignore or dismiss his or her own emotions, or express them in unhealthy or irresponsible ways. These behaviors can arrest the development of a child's affective self/other understanding and foster a negative attitude toward having and expressing certain feelings. Moreover, children who do not have good affective role models are often found to experience difficulties attuning their affects in line with the context and/or addressing the cause of their feelings. Regrettably, developmental shortcomings in this regard often lead to unhealthy behavior patterns in adult life, and a vicious cycle is established. Affect phobia can, however, also have sociocultural roots. We may, for instance, live in a society or work in an environment where feelings, such as sadness or anger, and their accompanying expression, are seen as a sign of weakness or lack of self-control. In certain cultural environments, the expression of emotions may even be perceived as offensive. These sorts of social pressures can impede the development of a healthy affective attitude.

Studies in the fields of attachment theory, affect regulation, mentalization and other related fields show that experiencing affects, including expressing and addressing them appropriately, is vital to our overall health and well-being. Suppressed feelings are often manifested in other feelings or behavior, such as tension, intrusive thoughts, or erratic behavior. A fear of affect disconnects us from ourselves and from the world around us, and it impedes our willingness and ability to affectively mentalize about ourselves and others. In a series of published research findings (see, for instance, McCullough, 1997; McCullough & Andrews,

2006), American psychotherapist Leigh McCullough, described a therapeutic model to deal with affect phobias. "Affect phobia therapy" focuses on the internal conflict patients experience regarding their affective mental states. To illustrate the conflict, anger may activate anxiety, which then activates some defense mechanism aimed at avoiding or inhibiting anger activation. Let us move on to an exploration of what affect entails.

Affect

"Affect" is defined by the online *APA Dictionary of Psychology* (2022) as "any experience of feeling or emotion, ranging from suffering to elation, from the simplest to the most complex sensations of feeling, and from the most normal to the most pathological emotional reactions." Affect is often described in terms of positive affect or negative affect. It relates to the composite of both *valence,* the intrinsic goodness or badness of an event, object, or situation, and *arousal.* Feelings, moods and emotions all comprise affect. Whereas affect is the *sensorial experience* we have, emotions, feelings and moods can be viewed as *personalized affect.* We describe our feelings when we want to understand and label sensations based on our own experiences. A mood, on the other hand, is a person's specific state of mind that generally lasts longer than an emotional expression, and is not readily associated with a specific cause. A mood can apply not only to people, but also to movies, music and other forms of entertainment or art. Emotions, in contrast, are the social expressions that help us communicate the way we feel to the outside world. We use emotions as a means of communication and to influence the behavior of others around us. Unlike moods, emotions are generally not long-lasting, and are much more readily associated with a specific elicitor. Of the four elementary mental states, affect is the mental state we can most easily observe directly, albeit predominantly with regard to basic emotional states such as anger and fear. Against this backdrop we will proceed to examine the concept of affect in relation to mentalization.

Important Social Functions of Expressing Emotions

The expression of emotions in the course of human interaction serves a number of important social functions. Drawing from studies on evolution, it appears that affective communication evolved in a social context, indicating that it must have been beneficial for social survival. Emotional expressions act as signals and cues from which we can infer how people affectively experience situations, or by which we recognize their attempt to influence the mental states and behavior of others. Affective mentalizing involves the conscious reflection upon, and understanding of, emotional expressions, and the inferential value those expressions have when it comes to ascertaining our own affective mental states and those of others. These inferences allow us to navigate emotionally charged situations and adjust our behavior to rebalance our own affective states and the affective states of others. In addition, affective mentalizing focuses on relational goals. These goals are directly related to maintaining healthy relationships.

With regard to mentalization in general, humans have two main relational goals during social interaction:

1. To affiliate and cooperate in order to establish and maintain social relationships with others.
2. To socially distance and compete in order to establish or maintain a desirable social position relative to others (e.g., social distancing from others who are deemed to have a lower status, or competing with others for coveted relational ties in order to maintain or gain status).

The ability to affiliate and cooperate with others, or to socially distance from or compete against others, requires complex affective thinking, which is a crucial component of strategic mentalizing, where we use this affective information to predict or explain behavior. Affective mentalizing focuses on the reciprocal sharing of "real-time" affective mental states in order to establish and maintain a healthy relationship during interactions with others, and to keep mentalization faculties online when situations become emotionally charged. Affective mentalizing cultivates a positive attitude toward dealing with emotional experiences and expressions. This, in turn, motivates us to improve our proficiency at sending and receiving affective messages. Affective mentalizing, for instance, helps us to determine the right level of assertiveness to use when we do not feel as though others are treating us fairly or with appropriate respect. It is often unfamiliarity with a particular feeling or emotion, coupled with the fear of losing control, or being thought of poorly by others, that keeps us from developing our affective understanding and affective regulation skills. As mentioned in the introductory paragraph of this chapter, these impediments are often linked to our cultural, social and familial upbringing, and the customs and habits that we have been exposed to.

Mentalizing About Basic Personal Affects

There are many layers to an affective experience. Affective mentalizing focuses on affective mental states and the interpersonal social aspects of affect. We are going to take a look at the different social affects that we can experience during our interactions with others. But first, we want to introduce you to some basic concepts concerning affects. When we think about affects, "basic emotions," such as happiness, surprise, fear, anger, disgust, contempt and sadness spring to mind. These basic emotions are the easiest to detect, as they can be observed directly via facial expressions and, to a lesser extent, body posture and movements. Generally speaking, however, we rarely deal exclusively with a discrete emotion, or observe a clear expression of that emotion. Sadness, for example, can be expressed in a number of different ways in addition to a sad face. Those expressions, in turn, may be susceptible to different interpretations. For instance, crying can signify sadness, but it can also indicate great relief or happiness. Basic emotions are often combined to form "complex emotions." For example, anger and disgust toward another person combine to form the affect of contempt. The more complex the affective behavior, the greater the need to rely upon indirect indicators to infer what is going on in the mind of another. Emotions are not only complex, they are also multidimensional and subject to change. We have a tendency to read primarily the emotions that are *most easily observed,* overlooking more subtle, but equally indicative, affect indicators. Moreover, we tend to relate the cause of an emotion to the object that is *most salient.* Therefore, we must learn to assess and deal with both readily observable and more latent emotional displays, and consider direct and indirect underpinnings for these emotions. Often, we need to rely upon verbal accounts to understand the complexity of the experienced emotions. *Gathering all the relevant observable and verbal affect signals and cues, and interpreting them accurately,* is the essence of affective mentalizing.

During affective mentalizing, it is helpful to separate primary emotions from secondary (or reactive) emotions. "Primary emotions" are emotions that we feel in connection with the eliciting source of the emotion. "Secondary emotions" are emotions that we feel about those primary emotions. By way of illustration, feeling anxious about an upcoming examination would be a primary emotion. Feeling irritated about the anxious feeling itself would be a secondary emotion. Secondary emotions can turn primary emotions into complex reactions. Secondary emotions may manifest as defense mechanisms against primary emotions, such as feeling ashamed for showing sadness, or feeling guilty for displaying anger. The ability to differentiate between primary and secondary emotions provides us with a fuller affective understanding. Secondary emotions are closely linked to mental time travel, our capacity to place ourselves mentally in events in the past, the present situation, or possible future scenarios. Secondary emotional reactions might be related to past experiences and assumptions about the world based on those experiences. They can also be related to our "real-time" self-identity appraisals, to our discomfort regarding the primary emotions we are experiencing, or to opinions about the people with whom we are dealing. Finally, secondary emotions can relate to affects concerning projections of possible future events. For instance, laughing at someone's misfortune can make people feel uncomfortable when they consider how they would feel under similar circumstances.

In addition, we need to distinguish between context congruent and context *in*congruent emotional expressions and affective experiences. When we sense that emotional expressions are not congruent with the situation, there might be more to a reaction than meets the eye. Generally, however, it is our expectation of how a person should react that creates confusion and incongruity. Affective mentalizing helps to fill in the gaps, as it requires us to gather additional information from an objective and nonjudgmental perspective. As previously mentioned, we need to account for intero- and exteroceptive sensations, which can impact the intensity of our emotional reactions. For instance, underlying factors such as fatigue, hunger or irritation, can exacerbate primary and secondary emotions and feelings.

Mentalizing About Social Affects

How do basic personal affects relate to interpersonal social affects? All emotions, including basic emotions, are social in the sense that we use them to navigate our interactions with others, to send interpersonal messages, and to provide intrapersonal signals about our own well-being and our appraisals of the world around us. In contrast to basic affects, which come to us more or less instinctively, social affects are particularly dependent upon agreements and conventions within our social reality. Basic emotions require no more than an awareness of *one's own physical state*. Social affects, on the other hand, depend upon the *thoughts, feelings, or actions of other people as well as sociocultural norms*. We know much less about social affective displays because they do not seem to map clearly to specific facial or vocal expressions. Some emotions, such as embarrassment or shame, are more social, as they would lose much of their meaning in the absence of another person to observe and react to them. Other social emotions linger on well after the social interaction is over, for instance, the feeling of guilt that persists when reflecting on a past transgression.

Owing to its social embeddedness, affective mentalizing is closely linked to the development of social affects. These affects developed in an evolutionary manner to enable people to *affiliate* and *cooperate* with one another, for example, to find a mate and raise children, or to work together with other group members to provide protection and improve the chances of finding food. In addition, social affects evolved to *strengthen competition* with outsider groups over access to resources, or among group members over status within the group. Finally, social affects evolved to *socially distance* from those who transgress social rules, undermine social cohesion, or increase the vulnerability of the group to external threats. Affective behavior that indicates social distancing, such as anger and disgust, is expressed to make transgressors feel socially isolated and vulnerable to dangers that are ameliorated by group protection. Social distancing is initially an attempt to reform the behavior of transgressors so that they can be included in the social group again.

Building upon the assertions of Jonathan Haidt (2003), social affects can be divided into self-conscious affects and moral affects. The category of "self-conscious affects," also called "self-evaluative emotions," is composed of a variety of social affects that relate to our sense of self and our consciousness of the reactions of others to us. Examples of self-conscious affects include embarrassment, guilt, shame, jealousy, envy, arrogance and pride. "Moral affects" comprise a category of social affects that overlap with self-conscious affects. Moral affects moderate the link between moral standards and moral behavior. Moral affects are comprised of affects that relate to the condemnation of others, such as contempt, anger and disgust. In addition, moral affects include affects related to the suffering of others, such as compassion, as well as affects related to praising others, such as gratitude and adulation. Moral affects pertain to the "feeling" part that helps us form and communicate moral judgments and decisions. These affects motivate behavioral responses based on social moral standards. Scholars who study moral emotions have proposed that this category of social emotions is crucial to understanding why people either adhere to or deviate from moral standards. "Moral affects provide the motivational force—the power and energy— to do good and to avoid doing bad" (Tagney et al., 2007, p. 347). Affective mentalizing is critical for strategic mentalizing, where we make moral judgments about others so that we can make better decisions about our affiliation with or avoidance of others. It is essential to scaffold our own moral behavior on the basis of positive moral behavior that others around us display, so that we will be well integrated within society.

Finally, the idea that affects have social functions does not imply that they are always socially desirable. Affects like anger, jealousy and contempt, but also love, happiness and pride, can become socially dysfunctional when they are too strong or out of control. Such affects may irreparably damage relationships, undermining the goal of achieving social adjustment or respected social standing.

The Impact of Affects on Mentalization

There are additional reasons we need to monitor affective states in the course of social interaction. As discussed previously, intense feelings and emotions can impact our ability to mentalize. This seems to be especially true in relation to strategic mentalizing. Let us examine how this works.

When considering the impact of affect on mentalization, the affect infusion model is instructive. The "affect infusion model" is a theoretical model developed by social psychologist Joseph Paul Forgas (1995). A key assertion of the model is that the impact of affect on critical thinking, including the processes of mental state reasoning, tends to be exacerbated in complex situations that demand substantial cognitive processing. Complex social interactions present the greatest need for high-level mentalization. In other words, when interactions become more complex, confusing and unpredictable, affect becomes more prominent in influencing our evaluations and responses. Forgas defined the term affect infusion as "the process whereby affectively loaded information exerts an influence on, and becomes incorporated into, the judgmental process, entering into the judge's deliberations, and eventually coloring the judgmental outcome" (Forgas, 1995). Strategic mentalizing, the highest level of mentalization, involves the highest level of complex cognitive processing, and therefore is most susceptible to the influence of emotions, feelings and moods. The most likely reason that strategic mentalizing is "infused" by affect, is because it involves all stages of critical thinking that enable people to reach an understanding of the mind. Affect can influence each stage in the cognitive processes of attention, decoding, inferring, associating and predicting or explaining. Affective mentalizing is, therefore, crucial to keeping our emotions, feelings and moods in check, thereby decreasing the risk of misguided theory of mind inferences.

Most social interactions cannot be fully understood without taking affective influences into account, although not everybody processes and understands affect at the same level. For instance, whereas some people have a hard time understanding the affective mental states of others, other people find it hard to understand their own affective mental states. In fact, it is not uncommon for the same person to suffer both difficulties. In severe cases, this can point to psychological and/or physiological conditions. These are characterized by subclinical inabilities to detect, identify and/or describe emotions in the self, or by difficulty in distinguishing and appreciating the emotions of others. Alexithymia, a disorder discussed in the section on basic mentalizing, is a clear example of such a condition. More often, however, the difficulties stem from a lack of practice, a lack of motivation, or both.

There are three key "*intra*personal" factors that influence a person's willingness and predisposition to affectively mentalize: the first factor relates to the person's attitude toward affective experience and emotional expression; the second factor relates to the level of affective knowledge and understanding that the person has about other people in general; and the third factor relates to the person's level of affective self-knowledge and understanding. Let us take a closer look at each of these factors starting with attitude toward affect.

Attitude Toward Affect

Research shows that our attitude toward affect significantly impacts our willingness and motivation to understand ourselves and others on an affective level. Attitude can be defined as a predisposed way of thinking or feeling about events, ideas, people, etc. Attitude is shaped by the evaluation a person makes about the subject of the attitude. Attitude toward affect is a complex mental state based upon a combination of the primary mental states of affect, desire, belief and knowledge about affect, such as:

- Positive or negative affects about experiencing and expressing emotions, moods and feelings, resulting in a judgment about their pleasantness or unpleasantness.
- A desire to share or to avoid the sharing of affective states.
- Beliefs about the importance of sharing affective experiences and expressions.
- Knowledge of the appropriateness or inappropriateness of affective experiences.

Judgments underlying our attitudes toward affect are shaped by a person's past (i.e., upbringing) and present (i.e., prevailing social attitudes).

The affect regulation strategy that different people employ has a lot to do with their attitude toward affect. Research indicates that our personal attitude toward affect predicts our preference for specific forms of affect regulation. Some strategies are less beneficial than others. Choosing the wrong strategy can even be destructive. One would assume that all people would logically select the best possible affect regulation strategy, but this is not necessarily the case. For instance, although research shows that it is better to actively deal with affective states than to suppress them, many people choose avoidance as their preferred strategy. This can be due to an upbringing or sociocultural background that shapes a person's attitude toward affect. In some cultures, for instance, it is normal for a person to express grief over a death in a particularly demonstrative way. In other cultures, expressions of sadness are discouraged, and consequently, cultural members do their best to conceal such feelings. Furthermore, a person's negative attitude toward affect could influence other people to avoid emotional expressions in that person's presence. This will be more evident as we now begin to explore the relationship between attachment theory and affective attitude.

The Relationship Between Attachment Theory and Affective Attitude

Attachment theory, first developed by John Bowlby and further extended by Mary Ainsworth (Bretherton, 1992), provides a particularly useful model for explaining differences in mentalization in general, but especially in regard to affective mentalizing and affect regulation. Attachment theory addresses a specific aspect of the way human beings respond to others during social interactions. These social responses often follow a consistent cognitive, affective and behavioral pattern based on an internal working model. An "internal working model" is a cognitive framework that is influenced by the early childhood experiences we have with our primary caregivers, and is used to interpret and guide our relationships later in life (e.g., Bretherton, 1997; Bretherton & Munholland, 1999). Internal working models originate in an individual as a result of early childhood interactions, especially interactions with important caregivers, who are responsible for accommodating the development of mentalization competencies and affect regulation. These early developed internal working models can have a lifelong impact on a wide range of social interactions, as they influence our mental states in general, including complex mental states such as attitude toward affect. Attachment theory is based on the notion that the evolutionary survival instinct of an infant drives its desire to stay close to its caregiver. Based on the interactions that a young child has with its caregiver, the child will adopt strategies to promote close proximity with the caregiver.

These strategies are incorporated into an internal working model that becomes the blueprint for the child's attachment relationships later in life. If the care and support provided by the caregiver is consistent, the child is likely to develop a secure attachment style. A child who receives inconsistent caregiver support is likely to develop an insecure anxious attachment style. If a child is deprived of caregiver support during early childhood, an insecure-avoidant attachment style will most likely develop. Bartholomew and Horowitz (1991) added a fourth attachment style, which they called insecure "disorganized," or "anxious/avoidant" attachment style. Children with this attachment style demonstrate elements of both *anxious* and *avoidant* attachment styles. The different attachment styles in relation to the view people hold of themselves and others, and in relation to their mentalization abilities and affective regulation competencies, can be described as follows:

- A **"secure" attachment style** is found in people who hold a positive view of themselves and others, and who possess well-developed mentalization abilities and affect regulation competencies.
- An **"insecure-anxious" attachment style** is found in people who have a negative view of themselves and a positive view of others. Their affect regulation competencies are often underdeveloped and their affective responses are likely to be influenced heavily by the conduct of those with whom they interact. Their mentalization efforts are often centered on their interactional partner rather than on themselves, and most likely are biased due to their anxious feelings.
- An **"insecure-avoidant" attachment style** is found in people who have a positive view of themselves, but a negative view toward others. Such people often present with affect regulation competencies that are well-developed, but rigidly applied. These people are less likely to apply much effort when it comes to mentalizing about others, however, when they do mentalize about others their inferences will most likely be biased due to their negative view of others.

- An "**insecure-disorganized" attachment style** is found in people who have an unstable, fluctuating, or confused view of themselves and others. Such people display elements of both anxious and avoidant attachment behavior in an inconsistent manner. These fluctuations are also reflected in their mentalization efforts, and in their affect regulation strategies.

The behavioral strategies grounded in the latter three attachment styles can be associated with fight, flight and freeze reactions that are often manifested when interactions go awry. It is not necessarily the case that someone with an unhealthy attachment style will exhibit the same response pattern under all circumstances. For instance, different interactional partners can arouse different internal working models (concomitant with the accompanying cognitive, affective and behavioral patterns).

Analogous to attachment styles, attitudes are *circularly linked* through their accompanied behavioral expressions. Our attitudes toward affect and the way we deal with emotions, feelings and moods are shaped by interactions with others, especially interactions that we have as children with our direct caregivers. These interactions either increase or decrease our desire and capacity to understand our own affective mental states and the affective mental states of others. Consequently, our attitude toward affect, either positive or negative, will be strengthened, and we will deal with our own and other's affective experiences in consonance with these attitudes. Recognizing this dynamic is the first step toward improving our affective mentalizing capabilities and avoiding unhealthy circular behavioral patterns. Once we truly grasp this concept, we can consciously choose the kind of attitude toward affect that promotes our understanding of, and connection with, others. People who fail to recognize and understand affects are often surprised by events, and tend to shun accountability for outcomes, leading to dysfunctional interpersonal interactions. That being said, most people do have a positive attitude toward affect, and a natural desire to understand themselves and others.

Based, in part, on our attitude toward affect, we make predictions about what is going to happen and how we and other people will feel about the event. This is a form of affective forecasting. "Affective forecasting" is the prediction of affect in the future. These predictions influence our willingness and motivation to approach or avoid situations, and our inclination to engage with some people but not with others. We make predictions about the valence (emotional force or attraction) of our future feelings, the specific affects that will be experienced, the intensity of these affects and their likely duration. Although research on affective forecasting with regard to others is scant, there are studies that show we do make empathic forecasts that include affective forecasts about other people. We do this especially for people whom we expect to encounter in our imagined future scenarios. This affective forecasting about ourselves and others prepares us for how to behave in these possible future encounters. Moreover, it is closely linked to affective theory of mind reasoning, upon which we base our predictions with regard to intentional and strategic behavior. Affective forecasting can, however, also bias our strategic predictions. People are fairly accurate when it comes to predicting affect in straightforward encounters, especially positive encounters. Research indicates, however, that affective forecasting becomes increasingly inaccurate with more complex or negative social encounters. We tend to *overestimate* the intensity and/or duration of the impact that an emotional event will have on our own future affective state, and on the future affective states of others. This is known as "impact bias." Affective forecasting can become a self-fulfilling prophecy in that our predictions about how we and others are going to feel in response to an event tend to influence the behavior we choose to apply in preparation for and during those events. This can result in our expectations coming to fruition. The affect infusion model described earlier in this chapter explains this impact of affect on critical thinking. Mentalization is critical to the accurate prediction of events, and affective forecasting is an important part of mentalization. As a situation unfolds, however, we need to maintain an open mind and monitor the *actual* progression of the encounter, recognizing that it could follow several different courses. Real-time mentalization needs to be grounded in nonjudgmental acceptance of what is actually happening. This enables us to remain attentive to new input and keep our mentalization faculties online, so that our inferences are not biased by "premeditated" affective states.

As previously discussed, different people have different attitudes toward affect. At one end of the spectrum are people who largely ignore emotions, often based on the attitude that affects should not play a prominent role in most day-to-day activities. These people tend not to confront their feelings, which they view as merely disruptive and upsetting. They prefer instead to employ coping mechanisms such as denial and avoidance. This behavior is frequently observed in people who demonstrate an insecure-avoidant attachment style. Many of the clinical psychological disorders - such as social anxiety disorder, borderline personality disorder and narcissism - involve unhealthy affective attitudes and responses. At the other end of the spectrum are people who take emotions into account in every aspect of their lives. They view emotions as conveying valuable information that helps them to navigate their way through life. For people falling at this end of the spectrum, social interactions without emotions would be flat and insipid. Provided these people have well-developed affect regulation competencies, this attitude toward affect is often demonstrated by people with a secure attachment style.

This concludes our discussion of affective attitude and its impact on affective mentalizing. We now turn to the second intrapersonal factor that impacts our motivation and ability to engage in affective mentalizing: our understanding of affective mental states.

Affective Understanding

Our understanding of affective states, their causes and impacts, is influenced by the fact that we are more inclined to share our own affective states, and accurately read the affective states of others, when:

- we feel comfortable with the particular emotional aspects, or in other words, when they belong to our own emotional repertoire;
- they are straightforward and salient; and
- they are consistent and appropriate given the context.

In addition, we are more motivated to deal with affects that are easy to share, such as sadness or anger, than complex affects, such as envy or jealousy. This might be related to our tendency to "embody" affects such as sadness or anger more readily, as a consequence of mimicry and affective contagion. Hence, people are simply better at reading and communicating emotions with which they are more comfortable, and those that are straightforward and easy to share. During social interaction, especially in situations that are, or can become, emotionally charged, regular monitoring of our own affective mental states and those of others is required. If we can quickly and accurately detect changes in affective mental states, we will be better able to defuse emotionally charged situations, restore equilibrium and assure that all parties concerned are taking one another into account. As we try to understand the affective reactions of other people, we also need to consider indirect external and internal factors, particularly when emotional reactions appear to be incongruent with the circumstances. For instance, nonsocial affective influencers (exteroceptive and interoceptive sensations) such as irritation or fatigue can exacerbate or diminish an emotional reaction. Indirect affective influencers can also be grounded in social concerns, such as fear of rejection. Making sense of social encounters requires proper *detection*, *processing* and *interpretation* of the affective mental states of others. Complex interactions often require an extra degree of inquiry and validation in order to clarify the meanings of affective mental states and to verify our inferences. Armed with an accurate and comprehensive affective assessment, we can identify and reconcile differences in the way participants view or experience a situation affectively, and gain better insight into ourselves and others.

Mentalizing about our own affective mental states entails the ability to recognize our own emotions, moods and feelings, coupled with the ability to associate those affects with their root causes. Improving our affective self-knowledge and understanding provides us with a greater sense of self-determination and a positive attitude toward affective experiences, leading to the enhancement of our affective mentalizing motivation and skill. People differ widely in how they reflect on their own feelings. To illustrate, people generally use two distinct kinds of information to diagnose their own affective states: *self-produced signals* and *situational cues.* When using self-produced signals, people rely on their own affect indicators, which are influenced by their own perceptions and emotional expressions. In contrast, when using situational cues, people rely on contextual factors to assess what they "must" be feeling, as judged by what they think other people in general would feel in a similar situation. People who associate emotions with their own affective "sensations," as opposed to situational cues, will be more likely to reflect on their own affective disposition, putting them in a better position to discover healthy ways of regulating their affective states. Affective intrapersonal mentalizing helps us to understand why we think, feel and behave in a certain fashion. This affective self-understanding presents us with the opportunity to explain our affective experiences to others. This is crucial if we want to elicit the right support or behavioral change from others, or to help others understand why our reaction may have seemed out of character. In addition, affective self-understanding is necessary to construct an accurate affective forecast of how we are likely to feel in a future scenario. As previously explained, our level of proficiency in predicting our own emotions has an impact on our behavioral decision-making. The course of action that we choose will, in turn, promote or diminish particular emotional consequences. Attaining greater insight into our own affective makeup allows us to make better behavioral decisions, which in turn enable us to better regulate how we experience situations affectively.

Accurate mentalizing about our own affective states, in turn, requires a well-developed affective self-understanding. This dynamic can be viewed as a *positive feedback loop,* whereby affective intrapersonal mentalizing and affective self-understanding increasingly strengthen each other. Research has indicated that the brain regions involved in gaining an understanding of others are also largely involved in gaining self-understanding. Accordingly, researchers have suggested that, to a certain extent, *we learn about others in essentially the same way that we learn about ourselves.* One important difference is that we have more information about ourselves than we have about others. The fact that we possess more information about ourselves does not necessarily mean, however, that we always have a well-developed self-understanding. Many studies have shown that people often have an inaccurate image of themselves. When people are asked to rate themselves on various personality traits, for instance, the big five - "open mindedness," "conscientiousness," "extraversion," "agreeableness," "neuroticism" - their ratings correlate *moderately* with the ratings that friends and family members give them. Is it possible to gain a truly accurate affective self-understanding? Studies aimed at measuring increases in self-understanding following self-awareness exercises indicate that it is definitely possible to improve the accuracy of our affective self-image. We now continue with a discussion of the key advantages, impediments and avenues for enhancement of affective attitude and affective understanding.

Improving Attitude and Understanding Regarding Affect: Advantages, Impediments and Avenues for Enhancement

ADVANTAGES

There are a number of advantages to having a positive attitude toward affect and a well-developed affective understanding. On an intrapersonal level, research shows that when we have a positive attitude toward affect, *we are more at ease in dealing with our own affective states.* A positive attitude toward affect also *helps us to remain vigilant of the impact that our own affect has on our own perceptions and judgments.* Recognizing that our attitude toward affect is shaped by our experiences, both past and present, empowers us to uncover the origins of unhealthy attitudes. This understanding further enables us to choose the kind of attitude toward affect that we want to embrace, and adjust any personal behavioral patterns that do not reflect our desired attitude. A positive attitude toward affect also *strengthens our motivation to develop a good understanding of our own affective makeup, our temperament, personality traits and affective style* (the manner in which we react to emotional situations). A well-developed affective self-understanding *helps us to apply complex affective thinking about ourselves.* Complex affective thinking enables us to comprehensively and accurately mentalize about our affective mental states. Only with this comprehensive affective understanding are we able to choose the right strategies for affect regulation. All these factors work together to reinforce a positive feedback loop: Affective understanding promotes a positive attitude toward affect, a positive attitude toward affect promotes affective mentalizing, and affective mentalizing increases affective understanding. Not surprisingly, this cycle applies equally to both affective self-understanding and affective understanding of others.

On an interpersonal level, a positive attitude toward affect *strengthens our motivation to improve our affective understanding of others and our affective understanding in general.* A better affective understanding of others increases our ability to view situations from the perspectives of others. It also enables us to apply complex affective thinking in order to better connect and cooperate with others. Affective mentalizing provides us with greater insight into how our own affective make up and style can impact others, and vice versa. These insights guide us in how to deal with, and help others deal with, emotionally charged situations. They also help us to better regulate our own reactions and to bring about the reactions we want to see from other people. As we will discuss in the next chapter, a positive affective attitude and well-developed affective understanding inspire us to empathize with, and show compassion toward, others.

On an extrapersonal level, affective understanding *helps us to detect sociocultural differences in affective processing and affective display rules*, and be conscious of how they impact our interactions with others on an intercultural level. This sort of intercultural affective acumen is a critical asset, as our range of interactions with others becomes increasingly diverse due to social media and globalization of work environments.

IMPEDIMENTS

There are also a number of impediments to developing a positive attitude toward affect and increasing our affective understanding. On an intrapersonal level we have seen that *having a negative attitude toward affect inhibits our affective development.* A negative attitude toward affect deprives us of opportunities to learn from our feelings and to understand ourselves affectively, leaving our affective world as largely uncharted territory with unanticipated pitfalls whenever our usual affective state is disrupted by significant events or emotionally charged experiences. A lack of affective awareness creates distance between us and others, as they have a hard time reading us on an affective level and vice versa. This unawareness impedes us from choosing the right environment in which to thrive, or the right people who can help us maintain healthy affective states. A negative attitude toward affect makes us feel out of control and leads us to say things like "*This just isn't me*" or "*I don't recognize myself.*" Such thoughts can make us feel overwhelmed and can influence us to fall back on superficial emotional management strategies, while foreclosing opportunities to learn something more about ourselves.

On an interpersonal level, *a limited affective self-understanding generally goes hand in hand with a limited affective understanding of others and a negative attitude toward sharing affective states*. We often pass our own negative attitudes on to others, particularly to children in our care, dampening their affective experiences and causing them to suppress their emotional displays. Not only is this an unhealthy way to deal with affects, but research has shown that it also deprives us of insight into the way others experience interactions or situations. It hinders our ability to detect affective mental states, a critical step in affective mentalizing. In addition, shortcomings in affective understanding tend to heighten empathic distress, making us self-focused and disrupting our capacity to mentalize about others. All of these factors feed into a negative attitude toward dealing with affective mental states. This negative feedback loop will be addressed in more detail in the upcoming chapter on empathy and compassion.

On an extrapersonal level, *sociocultural norms may dictate that individuals display affects that they do not truly feel, exaggerate displays of affect, or suppress expressions of emotions*. In such a social environment, a person has to engage in "emotion work" or "emotion management" in order to keep emotional displays in line with sociocultural rules. This can create a negative attitude toward particular affects and impede affective understanding. We need to take different affective sociocultural rules into account when integrating into new environments. Lack of familiarity with different affective sociocultural rules can lead us to overlook or misinterpret the meaning of affective behavior. Awareness of these differences, on the other hand, will alert us to the fact that we need to infer affective mental states from indicators other than, or in addition to, affective displays. Finally, if we are not familiar with, or fail to adhere to, the prevailing affective sociocultural rules, we can easily commit social faux pas. Now we will examine opportunities for fostering a positive attitude toward affect and improving our affective understanding.

AVENUES FOR ENHANCEMENT

Affective mentalizing is fundamental to the entire mentalization process, as it provides critical information about affective mental states and helps to keep our mentalization faculties online. In addition, it keeps our interactions and relations with others healthy and balanced. Affective mentalizing deficits can lead to a sense of affective helplessness. As previously discussed, studies indicate that this sort of affective distress may contribute significantly to psychological disorders, both minor and severe. Well-developed affective mentalizing skills and social competence are crucial to social interaction, as borne out by research on social isolation. Social isolation impedes the development of the very same mentalization and social intelligence competencies that we need to connect to, and sustain relationships with, others. Fostering a positive attitude toward affect and a better affective understanding requires us to take several measures. When it comes to affective attitude we need:

- To explore the affective mental states and emotional styles with which we feel comfortable, and those that make us feel uncomfortable.
- To examine the various relationships and situational contexts that impact our affective mental states, both positively and negatively.
- To discover the root causes of our discomfort and examine how we can replace old negative associations with positive new ones.

The insights that we gain from these measures will help to give us better command over our own affective attitude and behavior.

A positive affective attitude promotes an open-minded approach to developing good affective understanding of ourselves and others. Understanding the full breadth of affective experiences, especially those that are unfamiliar to us due to sociocultural differences in experiencing, expressing and dealing with affective states, is critical to mentalization, as it enables us to step away from our own perspectives and take the perspectives of other people into consideration.

Developing a comprehensive affective self-understanding requires that we examine and map all of the different aspects that constitute our affective makeup, such as:

- Temperamental predisposition.
- Personality traits.
- Affective style.
- Sensitivity with regard to exteroceptive and interoceptive stimuli.
- Affective thought and behavioral patterns with regard to particular people and situations.
- Affects with which we are comfortable and those that we would rather avoid.
- Strategic preferences we have for controlling and regulating affect.
- Affective differences from, and similarities to, other people from similar and dissimilar sociocultural environments.

We can develop a comprehensive affective understanding of others in the same way by mapping all of the different aspects that constitute their affective makeup.

Affective mentalizing teaches us to note and monitor the impact that our affective-state-influenced behavior has on others, and to evaluate our own affective reactions in relation to those of others. It bears repeating that *affective mentalizing is recursive in nature*. Done correctly, it fosters a positive feedback loop that continuously builds upon our self-understanding and our understanding of others.

We have defined affect, explained what affective mentalizing entails, and examined the factors that influence our motivation and ability to develop and apply our affective mentalizing competencies. In the next chapter, we discuss empathy and compassion in relation to affective mentalizing.

References

American Psychological Association. (n.d.). Affect. In *APA dictionary of psychology.* Retrieved July 17, 2022, from https://dictionary.apa.org/affect

Bartholomew, K., & Horowitz, L. M. (1991). Attachment styles among young adults: A test of a four-category model. *Journal of Personality and Social Psychology, 61*(2), 226–244. https://doi.org/10.1037/0022-3514.61.2.226

Bretherton, I. (1992). The origins of attachment theory: John Bowlby and Mary Ainsworth. *Developmental Psychology, 28(5), 759–775.* doi:10.1037/0012-1649.28.5.759

Bretherton, I. (1997). Bowlby's legacy to developmental psychology. *Child Psychiatry and Human Development, 28(1), 33–43.* doi:10.1023/a:1025193002462

Bretherton, I., & Munholland, K. A. (1999). *Internal working models in attachment relationships: A construct revisited.* In J. Cassidy & P. R. Shaver (Eds.), *Handbook of attachment: Theory, research, and clinical* applications (p. 89–111). The Guilford Press.

Forgas, J. P. (1995). "Mood and judgment: The Affect Infusion Model (AIM)". *Psychological Bulletin, 117*(1), 39–66. doi:10.1037/0033-2909.117.1.39

Haidt, J. (2003). *The moral emotions.* In R. J. Davidson, K. R. Scherer, & H. H. Goldsmith (Eds.), *Series in affective science. Handbook of affective sciences* (p. 852–870). Oxford University Press.

McCullough, L. (1997). *Changing Character: Short-term Anxiety-regulating Psychotherapy For Restructuring Defenses, Affects, And Attachment.* Basic Books.

McCullough, L., & Andrews, S. (2006). Assimilative Integration: Short-term Dynamic Psychotherapy for Treating Affect Phobias. *Clinical Psychology: Science and Practice, 8*(1), 82–97. doi:10.1093/clipsy.8.1.82

Tagney, J. P., Stuewig, J., & Mashek, D. J. (2007). "Moral emotions and moral behavior." *Annual Review of Psychology 58,* 345-72. doi:10.1146/annurev.psych.56.091103.070145

SECTION III.

AFFECTIVE MENTALIZING

To Simulate and Project

Chapter 2.

Empathy and Compassion

The Dark Triad

When we think of a person who is empathetic, we generally imagine a person who is kind and helpful. Empathy does not always have such a benevolent aim, however. There are people who are highly skilled at using their ability to empathize for selfish gain. These individuals often score significantly higher than average on scales that measure the Dark Triad. The "Dark Triad," a term coined by Paulhus and Williams in 2002, refers within the field of psychology to the personality traits of "psychopathy," "narcissism" and "machiavellianism." These three personality traits are together referred to as the Dark Triad because they share characteristics of a *callous-manipulative and selfish interpersonal style.* Although the jury is still out on whether these three personality traits are truly distinct personality constructs, research results on the Dark Triad are useful to explain how empathy should conjure up more than simply a benevolent image of an empathetic person.

Studies have noted certain common characteristics among the three personality constructs that make up the Dark Triad. As previously mentioned, manipulative behavior appears as a hallmark of all three constructs, although the way the manipulation manifests itself appears to vary significantly from one construct to the next. Jonason et al., in their 2012 research paper, concluded that all of the Dark Triad traits were associated with manipulation in the workplace, but each trait was driven by its own distinct mechanism. Machiavellianism, for instance, is associated with the use of manipulative, deceptive and immoral behavior to promote self-serving goals in callous disregard for any adverse impact on others. Individuals scoring high on the machiavellianism scale are often shrewd political players who do not shy away from the opportunity to exploit others for their personal gain. Being quick thinkers, they are able to use their manipulative strategies in a flexible way. In fact, Kowalski et al. (2001) found a significant positive correlation between machiavellianism and fluid intelligence. In the Jonason et al. study, machiavellianism was found to be especially associated with the use of excessive charm as an instrument of manipulation. Narcissism, the second personality construct of the Dark Triad, is characterized by a sense of grandiosity, vanity, pride and egotism. People who score high on the narcissism scale believe they are superior to others. They seek out opportunities to gain a lot of attention and praise from others. They bask in reflected glory by associating themselves with successful people and making it seem as though they played an important role in the success of those people. When narcissistic people feel that others are not feeding their inflated self-image, or are doubting their grandiosity, they can react aggressively and vengefully. In the Jonason et al. study, narcissism was closely associated with the use of physical appearance as an instrument of manipulation. Perhaps the darkest of the three Dark Triad constructs, psychopathy, an extreme form of antisocial personality disorder, is characterized by continuous antisocial behavior, impulsivity, selfishness, callousness and remorselessness. Individuals who score high on the psychopathy scale display impulsive and reckless behavior that often involves substantial risk. This risk may be physical, interpersonal, or financial. Psychopaths tend to be inflexible in their strategies and rather opportunistic. They are often identified by their disruptive interpersonal behavior, sometimes extending to sadistic behavior. This personality construct is often associated with deviant behavior and a criminal lifestyle. Psychopaths show high levels of recidivism, which may be related to a lack of regard for punishment. The Jonason et al. study found that psychopathy was particularly associated with physical threats as instruments of manipulation.

For many years it was assumed that people who score high on Dark Triad scales simply lacked empathy. As with manipulation, however, the atypical empathy scores common to all three personality constructs do not tell the whole story. There is a large body of research suggesting that all three personality constructs of the Dark Triad are characterized by atypical responses to distress cues, such as facial and vocal expressions of fear and sadness. While narcissism is not always characterized by such atypical responses, machiavellianism and psychopathy are. In their 2013 study, Jonason and Krause found that *high* scores on psychopathy, in particular, correlated with *low* scores on empathy. Recent research suggests, however, that these individuals do not truly lack empathy, but rather are *less sensitive* to certain emotional expressions, such as fear and anger. This lower sensitivity of psychopaths to the emotional expressions of others goes hand in hand with a high intrapersonal threshold to experiencing the same emotions. Psychopaths are therefore *less susceptible to affective contagion.* Other recent studies suggest, however, that a psychopath's atypical response to distress cues could be attributed to an inability to accurately map the expression of emotions by others, or their own sensations, to emotions such as fear or sadness. In other words, they do not *recognize* what they observe or sense as a particular emotion. In this sense, psychopaths appear to suffer from symptoms similar to individuals with alexithymia, a disorder discussed in the earlier chapter on basic mentalizing. In fact, a study by Cairncross et al. in 2013, indicated that there is a positive correlation between scores on psychopathy or machiavellianism and scores on alexithymia scales. This was not found to be the case with narcissism. Again, other research on psychopathy, such as that done by Meffert et al. in 2013, proposes that psychopaths are capable of empathizing, but they also have the ability to "switch these feelings off." A brain imaging study conducted by these researchers revealed that the initial difference between the control group and a group of psychopathic criminal offenders in empathic feelings for others was significantly reduced when the psychopaths were instructed to empathize with actors in video clips depicting emotional interactions. The Meffert et al. study suggests that empathy seems to be a *voluntary* activity for psychopaths. This might explain the ability of psychopaths to be charming and manipulative at the same time. Studies that measure empathy in relation to the Dark Triad are especially focused on affective empathy, the capacity to feel what others feel, as opposed to cognitive empathy, the capacity to imagine what others must be feeling under the circumstances.

How is it that psychopaths are able to switch their empathy on and off? Actually, theories on evolution suggest that we are all wired to resist empathizing with others. The ability to inhibit empathy presents clear evolutionary benefits. Our primal instincts of self-preservation and survival can easily suppress our empathy for others. To illustrate, if we feel threatened by a situation, our instinctive reaction to escape the threat may override our motivation to empathize with others who are exposed to the same threat. However, it is more natural for people in general to empathize with others than it is for psychopaths. Some people can experience empathic feelings that are so overwhelming they lead to empathic distress. Fortunately, people can hone their ability to inhibit the disruptive effect of empathic feelings through affective mentalizing techniques aimed at regulating empathic distress. Medical professionals, for instance, must learn to effectively deal with the empathy that they feel for their patients in order to stay focused on their work. Good mentalization practices are well-suited to improving our empathic regulation skills, as we will discuss later.

Psychological literature has provided us with new understandings of how individuals associated with the constituent personality constructs of the Dark Triad employ affective mentalizing solely as a means of gathering information to be used for strategic mentalizing inferences. For these individuals, social responses such as empathy and compassion for others do not come naturally. Their affective mentalizing about others is motivated instead by their own goal-directed intentions. It could be argued that these individuals actually skip or disregard the level of affective mentalizing by perceiving all affective input from a strategic mentalizing point of view. Consequently, in situations that are not of direct consequence to them, they probably fail to recognize the importance of critical affect indicators. But what if a situation is consequential to such a person? As previously discussed, these individuals have the ability to infer affective mental states and empathize with others in a benevolent way, provided they choose to do so. They do so, however, only when their failure to empathize would subject them to negative consequences, or when empathizing with others would further their own goals. Individuals associated with the Dark Triad are more likely to pick up on affect signals and cues in a *non*embodied way, in other words, i.e., as a "detached observer." Studies support the conclusion that these individuals employ *cognitive* empathy (i.e., the capacity to understand what others are feeling without actually feeling it). Individuals who score high on the Dark Triad scale do not try to feel what others are feeling (simulation). Instead, they imagine themselves in the shoes of others (projection), or they simply employ affect indicators that are useful for their own strategic purposes. In other words, they bypass much, if not all, of the affective mentalizing process. They gather affect signals and cues on a cognitive level, and combine them with other mental states such as beliefs and desires, to form rational models of what is going on in the minds of others. These mental state inferences may help them to cooperate with others, but only when it furthers their own goals, or to compete against others, often ruthlessly, if that appears to be a better option.

Does all of this make Dark Triad personalities better or worse at reaching accurate theory of mind inferences than the general population? Research suggests that these individuals are not universally at an advantage or disadvantage when it comes to reasoning about what is going on in the minds of others. To illustrate, when an understanding of affective states is needed in order to maintain a healthy relationship, they are inclined to neglect these states as their goal-directed intent outweighs their desire to maintain healthy relationships. They do not embody the way others feel, and are therefore less motivated to show compassion for others. Moreover, they do not feel remorse the way people do in general. This kind of callousness makes it easier for them to use affective information for their own benefit, and at the expense of others. At the very least, they are less distracted by the affective states of others, which keeps their strategic mentalizing faculties sharp. As a trade-off, however, they fail to mentalize in a way that helps them maintain healthy relationships with others. Coupled with the intelligence to use affective information strategically, Dark Triad personalities can be ruthless, even dangerous.

The Dark Triad has proven to be a highly useful concept when it comes to predicting and explaining antisocial behavior and extreme forms of competitive behavior that are devoid of affective mentalizing and its accompanying goal of maintaining healthy relationships with others. We have spent a fair amount of time examining personality traits that tend to inhibit a person's ability and motivation to empathize with others with benevolent intent. Now we will examine complementary attribute sets that promote prosocial behavior.

The Light Triad

Is there such a thing as a "Light Triad?" The research of Kaufman et al. (2019) is devoted to answering this question. These scholars devised a Light Triad scale to measure three personality constructs that stand in contrast to the Dark Triad. They formulated their three Light Triad personality constructs as follows:

1. "**Faith in humanity**," the belief that humans in general are good.
2. "**Humanism**," the belief that humans, across all backgrounds, are deserving of respect and appreciation.
3. "**Kantianism**," the belief that others should be treated as ends in and of themselves, and not as pawns in one's own game.

These personality constructs are not as identifiable in people as are the constructs that make up the Dark Triad. For instance, it is probably easier for most people to recognize psychopathic behavior in a person than it is to identify kantianism in a person. Interestingly, *the Light Triad is not simply the opposite of the Dark Triad*, as the total Dark Triad scores and total Light Triad scores demonstrated only a moderate negative correlation of -.48 (Kaufman et al., 2019). As Kaufman et al. describe "[i]t appears that at least in terms of personality, the absence of darkness does not necessarily indicate the presence of light. There also appears to be some degree of independence between the Light and Dark Triad, leaving room for people to have a mix of both light and dark traits." The conclusions of Kaufman et al. can be reconciled with the dual, and sometimes competing, objectives of mentalization: enhancing cooperation and gaining competitive advantage. To illustrate, attaining a positive social standing often requires *close cooperation* with others, which is well served by personality traits of the Light Triad. Improving one's social status, on the other hand, can also require *competition* with others, which implicates behavioral elements akin to those employed by people who score high on the Dark Triad scale, but confined to the boundaries of respectful and moral human conduct.

According to the research of Kaufman et al., individuals scoring higher on the Light Triad scale reported:

- higher levels of secure attachment style in their relationships,
- mature defense styles, and
- optimistic beliefs about the self, the world and one's future.

These study subjects were also described as less focused on achievement and self-enhancement, and more concerned with productivity and competence. In the same research, Kaufman et al. found that high scores on the Light Triad were significantly correlated with high scores on scales that measure empathy and compassion. Interestingly, they concluded that "[w]hile having such 'loving kindness' even for one's enemies is conducive to one's own well-being, these attitudes, coupled with greater interpersonal guilt, could make those scoring higher on the Light Triad potentially more open to exploitation and emotional manipulation from those scoring higher on the Dark Triad." Having explored the dark side and the light side of human behavior, we now proceed to examine the concepts of empathy and compassion in greater detail.

In the remainder of this chapter, we will map out the *progression from affective contagion and affect indicator processing to empathizing and acting compassionately*. We will examine the difference between two forms of empathy – "affective empathy" and "cognitive empathy" - and discuss the influence of empathic distress on compassionate behavior. Because empathy can be used with both benevolent and malevolent intent, it should not be mistaken for compassion. Acts of compassion are always aimed at alleviating the suffering of people. Compassion should be viewed as a next step that we can choose to take after empathizing with others. Compassion moves us beyond empathizing to sympathizing with the person in need, and responding to the person's concerns or feelings with benevolent intent.

Affective and Cognitive Empathy

"Empathy" is an aspect of affective mentalizing that involves interpreting the affect signals and cues we gather from others in order to ascertain their affective mental states. Derived from the Greek "empatheia" (literally translated as "in feeling"), empathy is defined in the online *APA Dictionary of Psychology* (2022) as "understanding a person from his or her frame of reference rather than one's own, or vicariously experiencing that person's feelings, perceptions, and thoughts. Empathy does not, of itself, entail motivation to be of assistance, although it may turn into sympathy or personal distress, which may result in action." Empathy is critical for affective mentalizing, as emotionally charged interactions can impede our capacity to mentalize and damage our relationships with others.

The evolutionary origins of the ability to empathize with others can be traced back to the evolution of our capacity for "mental time travel." We have already touched on the subject of mental time travel: the capacity to project oneself into situations in the past, into imagined alternative scenarios in the present, and into possible scenarios in the future. It is part of what we do when we engage in backward or forward chaining to explain past behavior or to predict probable future behavior. According to studies on mental time travel, our ability to travel backward in time evolved before our ability to travel forward in time. Tulving (1985), who coined the term "mental time travel," argued that our memory system related to remembering personal experiences (our episodic memory) allows for this backward and forward time travel. Schacter et al. explain in their 2007 article that "brain regions that have traditionally been associated with memory appear to be similarly engaged when people imagine future experiences." These researchers argued that "[g]iven the adaptive priority of future planning, we find it helpful to think of the brain as a fundamentally prospective organ that is designed to use information from the past and the present to generate predictions about the future." The "prospective brain," as described by Schacter et al. in the same article, is crucial for strategic planning and behavioral flexibility. Using mental time travel, we think of ourselves as alternate "selves" that can exist either in a past, present, future, or timeless imagined situation. In other words, people can simultaneously maintain multiple temporal perspectives. Analogously, Schacter et al. argue that "thinking about the perspectives of others (theory of mind) also appears to use the core brain system." In this case, however, we hold our own perspective, along with the perspectives of others, in our minds simultaneously, an ability we refer to as "perspective shifting." Both our concept of "self" and our capacity to empathize with others are dependent upon the ability to "split" ourselves off (affectively and behaviorally) from others. In our earlier chapter on basic mentalizing, we explained that affect and behavior are often shared subconsciously, through mimicry, affective contagion and behavioral contagion. Through these mechanisms, we experience shared affect and behaviors just as though they had emerged from within ourselves. As we have seen, this can lead to confusion, since we do not naturally consider the possibility that our own affects and behaviors could possibly have originated with others. Maintaining a proper self-other distinction is critical for the development of an accurate self-image, regulation of empathic distress, and empathetic and compassionate behavior toward others. Mental time travel is closely related to affective mentalizing. We can employ "empathic mental time travel" to deal with traumatic past events, respond appropriately to events in real-time and facilitate affective forecasting. There is yet another relationship between mental time travel and empathy. De Waal suggests in his 2008 article that empathy may have evolved as a proximate mechanism for altruism. Steinberg (2010) defines altruism as "intentional and voluntary actions that aim to enhance the welfare of another person in the absence of any quid pro quo external rewards." Associating with people who are reliable reciprocators of altruistic behavior provides an important survival benefit. Society thrives when everybody contributes to the public welfare through acts of altruism. In order for these recurring empathetic interactions to evolve, the ability for mental time travel, together with the capacity to form episodic memories, was essential. Only by remembering what tribal members did for each other in the past were early humans able to maintain a healthy balance in their reciprocal efforts, and to detect those who would cheat the system.

Research in cognitive neuroscience has identified the neural bases of two different forms of empathy, (Nummenmaa et al., 2008; Shamay-Tsoory, 2011). On the one hand, they found a strongly *embodied* form of empathy, referred to as "affective empathy." On the other, they found a strongly *cognitive* form of empathy, known as "cognitive empathy." Affective empathy evolved to strengthen fundamental bonds between humans and to promote altruistic behavior. In response to an increasingly complex social environment, cognitive empathy evolved in humans to provide a means of navigating more complex social interactions. Let us take a closer look at both of these empathic responses, beginning with affective empathy.

AFFECTIVE EMPATHY

"Affective empathy" involves "simulation," sharing in the full affective experience of another through mimicry and affective contagion. Simulation can be seen as the more basic form of empathy - a "bottom-up" strategy that requires the observer to detect and decode signals that are embodied and directly perceptible from interpersonal interaction. The social and nonsocial information derived from basic mentalizing mechanisms, involving the conscious processing of mimicry and affective contagion, supply us with the raw data that we need in order to empathize with others. Owing to the strongly embodied nature of mimicry and affective contagion, we can easily mistake the raw data as originating within ourselves. In order to truly empathize, however, we need to recognize that the information actually originated with others. In other words, this self-other distinction regarding the origin of sensations highlights the difference between mimicry and affective contagion on the one hand, and real empathy on the other. Affective empathy promotes our understanding of *what* others are feeling. Abnormalities in this form of empathy are common among people with alexithymia and those scoring high on the Dark Triad scales. To illustrate, research has associated psychopathy with a lower than normal sensitivity to the facial expression of fear. We now move on to cognitive empathy.

COGNITIVE EMPATHY

"Cognitive empathy" involves "self-projection," imagining one's self in the situation as another person, and projecting one's own feelings, thoughts and behaviors on that hypothetical scenario based on the assumption that the other must think and feel the same way. It consists of re-creating another's affective state within ourselves, based on our own affective perspective in relation to the other person's situation, in order to gain insight into the other's mental state. Contrast this with affective empathy, which relies on mimicry and affective contagion for mental state inferences. Cognitive empathy is a more advanced form of empathy, as it relies less on the decoding of signals from the immediate situation, and more on "top-down" strategies that require the use of mental representations formed in the observer's own mind. Cognitive empathy supports our understanding of *why* others feel the way they do. Hence, through cognitive empathy, we can infer the root-cause of another's feelings. Affective empathy and cognitive empathy provide us with different pieces of the puzzle that we can combine in order to make accurate affective mental state attributions. When people rely solely on *affective* empathy, they do not necessarily understand *how the feelings of others came about.* On the other hand, when people rely solely on *cognitive* empathy, they do not necessarily understand *what the other person truly feels.* True empathy flows from a combination of the distinctly separate mechanisms of affective empathy and cognitive empathy. Both affective and cognitive empathy can lead to the motivation to act compassionately. In contrast to cognitive empathy, however, affective empathy can more easily lead to empathic distress, which can impede the willingness to help others, as we will now discuss.

Empathic Distress

When we empathize with others we learn about their challenges and needs. Frequently, this understanding leads to a desire to alleviate the suffering of others through acts of compassion. This is not always the case, however. The roots of empathy are always initially self-focused, either because of the embodied sharing in another's affect, or the projection of one's self into the situation of another. The actual experience of empathy, however, subsequently becomes other-focused. As previously mentioned, our empathic disposition can vary from prosocial and altruistic to self-centered and ruthless. Some people find their empathetic feelings for others to be uncomfortable, or even overwhelming. This is called "empathic distress," an affective mental state characterized by the inability to endure the perceived pain or suffering of another person. Scientists propose that empathic distress often stems from a genetic predisposition. They also acknowledge, however, that a personal history of unresolved, sometimes traumatic, emotional events is almost always a principal factor underlying empathic distress. When we are in a state of empathic distress, we may experience the pain or emotion even more intensely than the other person does. This increases our self-focus and impedes the progression to "other-focused" empathy. We remain focused on alleviating our own empathic distress. Empathic distress can elicit "empathic anger" (anger about harmful consequences), feelings of injustice and guilt. As with any emotionally-charged or stressful situation, the experience of empathic distress can also paralyze our ability to mentalize. Our ability and our willingness to show compassion and support for others hinge on a number of factors in addition to empathic distress. For instance, they are strongly affected by the identity and behavior of the person who is suffering. *Is that person a stranger, or is it someone we know? Are we similarly situated? Does the person "deserve" it? How does the suffering of the person impact me?* Empathic distress, however, can be so overwhelming that we do not even begin to consider the other factors that mediate our ability and willingness to offer assistance before turning away from the person in need. This sort of strongly embodied sharing of distress - earlier referred to as affective empathy - can be especially challenging for healthcare workers, such as psychotherapists, physicians, or nurses. According to research, the best way to deal with empathic distress is to directly address the suffering of others. Empathic distress can also be alleviated through the employment of affect regulation strategies. Interestingly, research indicates that affect regulation is strengthened through self-compassion. Let us take a closer look at what compassion, including self-compassion, entails.

Other- and Self-Compassion

Compassion can be described as the concurrence of empathic concern together with a desire to help, and these mental states are often converted into prosocial behavior. Goetz and Simon-Thomas (2017) propose the following working definition of compassion: "a state of concern for the suffering or unmet need of another coupled with a desire to alleviate that suffering." They also mention the following constituent components of compassion:

- Awareness of the suffering or need of another.
- An affective state that motivates action.
- An appraisal of this state and whether offering help is possible regarding the (social) context.
- A judgment about the person who is suffering and the situational context.
- Engagement of the neural systems that drive social affiliation, cooperation and caregiving.

These components are not listed in any particular order and can often occur out of sequence. Looking at the Goetz and Simon-Thomas model, compassion can be viewed as a *complex* mental state that emerges from the primary mental states of affect, desire, belief and knowledge. To illustrate, we *feel* moved by the suffering of another, we *know* that we have the ability to help, we *believe* that the person deserves our help, and we have the *desire* to alleviate the hardship of the person who is suffering. In our previous discussion of empathy, we examined the difference between empathy and compassion. Whereas empathy involves our attempt to *understand* the suffering of others, compassion is aimed at *alleviating* that suffering. In contrast to affective empathy, compassion entails feeling *with* or *for* the other, and not merely feeling the same way the other person does. Nor should compassion be confused with cognitive empathy. As we have seen, cognitive empathy involves the process of *reaching an understanding* of the feelings of others through consideration of how we would feel in a similar situation. Compassion provides us with the motivation to *take action* to alleviate the perceived suffering. Empathic concern, on the other hand, even with benevolent intent, does not always evolve into compassionate behavior. Quite often, we first have to weigh the risk of taking action against our desire to alleviate suffering. We are evolutionarily wired to engage in this deliberation. To illustrate, when our ancestors went out to hunt big game, they needed to work together as a team to bring down a large animal. However, if the animal attacked one person in the group, the rest of the group had to consider whether to attend to their own (or the group's) safety, or help the victim of the attack. Often, we are not even aware that these competing instinctual forces are at work. Research on the "bystander effect," otherwise known as "bystander apathy," provides us with a better understanding of the reasons why we are not always moved to act with compassion, even when we can or should. The bystander effect pertains to the phenomenon that individuals are less likely to offer help to a victim when other people are present. Empathic distress turns out to be an important factor in the decision whether or not to act compassionately. Hortensius and De Gelder (2018) argue that "[i]n the presence of other bystanders, personal distress is enhanced, and fixed action patterns of avoidance and freezing dominate." We previously discussed two different ways to alleviate empathic distress: directly addressing the suffering of others and applying affect regulation strategies. We also noted that affect regulation was strengthened by self-compassion.

"Self-compassion" is defined by Neff (2003) as "being kind and understanding toward oneself in instances of pain or failure rather than being harshly self-critical; perceiving one's experiences as part of the larger human experience rather than seeing them as isolating; and holding painful thoughts and feelings in mindful awareness rather than over-identifying with them." We can apply self-compassion when we perceive ourselves as inadequate, when we are unsuccessful in our efforts, or when we experience general suffering. Self-compassion should be distinguished from "self-pity," which involves viewing oneself as a victim and lacking the ability to cope with an adverse situation. As with compassion for others, self-compassion is rooted in early attachment experiences, and is associated with maternal care, warmth and healthy family dynamics. A positive affective attitude and well-developed affective understanding are critical for empathy and compassion, as discussed in the previous chapter. Next, we will examine how empathy and compassion relate to affective mentalizing.

Empathy, Compassion and Affective Mentalizing

Let us start by examining what affective mentalizing encompasses. Affective mentalizing involves:

- Focusing in on affective mental states.
- Discerning the underlying feelings and the true origins of these feelings.
- Understanding that our feelings are in response to the emotional experience of another, not our own emotional experience.
- Understanding when empathizing is required.
- Being aware that we are empathizing.
- Recognizing the level on which we are empathizing (affective and/or cognitive).
- Purposefully progressing from mere empathy to compassion.
- Selecting and applying appropriate compassionate action.

Affective mentalizing sharpens our empathy and compassion practices through the conscious monitoring of our own affective mental states and those of others. It guides the entire process, from affect indicator detection to compassionate action. Affective mentalizing advances us beyond the initially observed affect indicators and our first impression of the cause for these feelings (information that we gather with our basic mentalizing skills). Affective mentalizing is needed to assure that we *empathize with the true feelings of others, and the underlying causes for those feelings*, in order to offer the compassionate assistance that is suited to their actual needs. At times, however, good affective mentalizing practices might militate in favor of exercising compassionate restraint out of respect for the privacy interests or the sociocultural rules that prevent others from revealing the true nature and cause of their emotions. We have already highlighted the importance of affective mentalizing to the processes of empathy and compassion. Empathy and compassion are equally important to the process of mentalization in general. Empathy and compassion are essential to keeping an open mind, remaining receptive to social information and promoting cooperation-based interaction. Studies in the field of neurology confirm that affective mentalizing is neurologically associated with both empathy and compassion. In their 2008 study, Hooker et al. found that cognitive empathy involved brain regions associated with mentalization and empathy. These researchers suggested that,

> there are many occasions in which the other person's emotional response is not observable but instead has to be inferred or imagined. These aspects of 'affective mentalizing' (or 'affective TOM') have not been adequately studied. Nonetheless, it is the ability to predict someone else's emotional response which provides the opportunity to use that affective representation to guide behavior in ways that prevent harm or promote well-being in others.

Hooker et al. also propose "that greater use of these affective representations when trying to understand the emotional experience of others is related to more empathy." They also found that "emotional empathic response is driven mainly by simulation and involves regions that mediate emotional experiences (i.e., amygdala, insula)." Relating mentalization to compassion, Allen et al. argue in their 2017 article that "[i]t is possible that the ability to accurately infer and reason about the mental state of others is a key psychological mechanism allowing individuals high in Compassion to behave in ways that foster greater cooperation and harmony within their relationships." These studies demonstrate the interrelated and interdependent connection between affective mentalizing and empathy and compassion. We now continue to the key advantages, impediments and avenues for enhancement of empathy and compassion practices in connection with affective mentalizing.

Cultivating Empathic and Compassion Practices: Advantages, Impediments and Avenues for Enhancement

ADVANTAGES

An enhanced understanding of empathy and compassion offers several key advantages. On an intrapersonal level, people with a well-developed sense of empathy and compassion *feel in control and at ease when faced with the distress of others,* and therefore are more willing and better equipped not only to provide support, but also to determine what precisely the other person needs. These people tend to be emotionally sensitive, creative and genuinely concerned for others, in a self-effacing way. Due to their willingness to empathize and show compassion, they engage more readily in situations where they can practice these skills. Self-compassion is important for both affective mentalizing and affect regulation, as it lowers levels of empathic distress and inhibits the emergence of a strong negative self-focus.

On an interpersonal level we see that *empathy supports affective mentalizing* by focusing our attention on the affect signals and cues that suggest the best course of action to alleviate suffering. Research indicates that the capacity for compassion significantly improves interpersonal relationships. Thus, empathy and compassion help us to maintain healthy relationships, keep our mentalization faculties online, and increase the accurateness of our affective mental state inferences.

On an extrapersonal level, research shows that those who have high levels of empathy, accompanied by low levels of empathic distress, are more likely to *function well in society, have larger social support groups and enjoy more satisfying social interactions and friendships.*

IMPEDIMENTS

There are also a number of factors that can impede our ability or willingness to empathize and show compassion. On an intrapersonal level, *we can be challenged by physical or psychological disorders that hinder our ability to empathize with others.* Such disorders may stem from a wide variety of conditions, such as a lack of emotional responsiveness to distress cues, an insensitivity to punishment and negative feedback, atypical socio-emotional information processing, or poor affect regulation skills. Given the complex nature of empathy, the causes and consequences of empathy impairments vary significantly. A low threshold for empathic distress also works against our capacity to empathize and show compassion. Empathic distress, in general, causes us to focus on ourselves and look for ways to escape the stressful situation. High levels of empathic distress are associated with a negative attitude toward affect and affective expressions along with a reticence to engage in compassionate behavior. In addition, limitations in complex affective thinking abilities can prevent people from reacting in an appropriately compassionate way. Finally, our mental state at any given time can impede our capacity to empathize or show compassion. To illustrate, when we feel tired or depressed, or when we are focused on ourselves or on our own goals, we do not have the mental bandwidth to deal with the suffering of others.

Interpersonally, *our motivation to empathize or show compassion can be influenced by our perception of the person in need.* People who are very different from us, whom we believe are to blame for their own suffering, or whom we think should be able to take care of themselves, are less likely to receive our empathic concern or compassion. Our motivation is likewise influenced by the relationship we have with the person in need. For instance, strangers and people whom we will never see again are less likely to receive our empathy and compassion than family members and friends. This is partly influenced by our implicit preference for dealing with reliable reciprocators.

On an extrapersonal level, *sociocultural circumstances can impede our motivation to empathize with others and to act compassionately toward them.* To illustrate, we sometimes hesitate to empathize and show compassion because we are not familiar with the prevailing sociocultural rules. In addition, *the situational context can make it impractical for us to lend a hand,* for instance, when we are not capable of providing the special care or assistance that is needed. The medium through which we communicate can also impede our ability to empathize and show compassion. When hardship is communicated only through written language - for instance via email - careful semantic processing may be necessary to mediate the connection between the feelings of the distressed person and the empathic response of the reader. This creates an "empathy gap." This gap can be narrowed through the use of emoticons that can act as surrogates for facial expressions or body language. Let us examine how we can improve our capacity for empathy and compassion.

AVENUES FOR ENHANCEMENT

We have seen that accurate empathizing depends on the ability to empathize on two levels:

1. Affective empathy, which involves feeling the same emotion as the other person as a step toward understanding what others are feeling.
2. Cognitive empathy, which involves reaching an understanding of the nature and cause of the affective mental state of others.

Together, these forms of empathy help us to gain a comprehensive and accurate perspective of the needs of others. Research indicates that both affective and cognitive empathy can be cultivated, and that people can learn to switch back and forth between the two. The ability to alternate between affective and cognitive empathy is critical to lowering empathic distress. Affective empathy can be bolstered by embodied training techniques, through which we can learn to simulate affective mental states in a controlled and regulated fashion in order to gain a more comprehensive empathetic understanding. Cognitive empathy can be enhanced via cognitive training techniques through which we can learn to project ourselves into affective mental states of others and to verify and discuss these projections in a manner that promotes empathetic understanding.

Reduction of empathic distress can be achieved by enhancing our affect regulation competencies. As previously discussed, affect regulation refers to the mental processes that work together in attending to, selecting and successfully monitoring and controlling thoughts, emotions and behaviors. Of course, these processes must entail a recognition of the origins of, and influences on, our own affective mental states.

While empathy training focuses on the detection and understanding of the suffering of others (and our own suffering), compassion training focuses on alleviating this suffering. Our capacity for compassion can be enhanced on two levels:

1. Compassion for others
2. Self-compassion

Learning to become more compassionate involves:

- Removing impediments to showing compassion.
- Developing effective communication strategies regarding:
    - How to approach people who are suffering.
    - Methods of soothing others and creating a safe environment.

  - Options for inviting others to join in compassionate acts when we need assistance or when we are not able to provide the necessary support.
  - Ways to say "no" in a compassionate way.
- Developing techniques to prevent compassion fatigue.
- Practicing self-compassion.

As with previous competencies, however, before we start looking at ways to enhance this component of affective mentalizing we need to *establish a baseline*. We determine this baseline by assessing our inclination for affective and cognitive empathy, our susceptibility to empathic distress, and affect regulation strategies we use to mitigate unhealthy levels of empathic distress, and our capacity for both self-focused and other-focused compassion.

The reflective nature of affective mentalizing sharpens our empathy and compassion practices through the conscious monitoring of our own affective mental states and those of others. It guides the entire process, from affect indicator detection, to affective resonance, to the recognition of that resonance as affective empathy, to an understanding of mental states achieved through cognitive empathy, and finally to the motivation to act compassionately.

References

Allen, T. A., Rueter, A. R., Abram, S. V., Brown, J. S., & Deyoung, C. G. (2017). Personality and neural correlates of mentalizing ability. *European Journal of Personality, 31*(6), 599–613. doi:10.1002/per.2133

American Psychological Association. (n.d.). Empathy. In *APA dictionary of psychology*. Retrieved July 17, 2022, from https://dictionary.apa.org/empathy

Cairncross, M., Veselka, L., Schermer, J. A., & Vernon, P. A. (2013). A Behavioral Genetic Analysis of Alexithymia and the Dark Triad Traits of Personality. *Twin Research and Human Genetics, 16*(03), 690–697. doi:10.1017/thg.2013.19

De Waal, F. B. M. (2008). Putting the altruism back into altruism: The evolution of empathy. *Annual Review of Psychology, 59*(1), 279–300. doi:10.1146/annurev.psych.59.103006.093625

Goetz, J. L., & Simon-Thomas, E. (2017). *The landscape of compassion: Definitions and scientific approaches.* In E. Seppala, E. Simon-Thomas, S. L. Brown, M. C. Worline, C. D. Cameron, J. R. Doty (Eds.), *The Oxford Handbook of Compassion Science* (pp. 3). Oxford University Press.

Hooker, C. I., Verosky, S. C., Germine, L. T., Knight, R. T., & D'Esposito, M. (2008). Mentalizing about emotion and its relationship to empathy. *Social Cognitive and Affective Neuroscience, 3*(3), 204–217. doi:10.1093/scan/nsn019

Hortensius, R., & de Gelder, B. (2018). From empathy to apathy: The bystander effect revisited. *Current Directions in Psychological Science, 27*(4), 249–256. doi:10.1177/0963721417749653

Jonason, P. K., Slomski, S., & Partyka, J. (2012). The Dark Triad at work: How toxic employees get their way. *Personality and Individual Differences, 52*(3), 449–453. doi:10.1016/j.paid.2011.11.008

Jonason, P. K., & Krause, L. (2013). The emotional deficits associated with the Dark Triad traits: Cognitive empathy, affective empathy, and alexithymia. *Personality and Individual Differences, 55(5),* 532–537. doi:10.1016/j.paid.2013.04.027

Kaufman, S. B., Yaden, D. B., Hyde, E., & Tsukayama, E. (2019). The light vs. dark triad of personality: Contrasting two very different profiles of human nature. *Frontiers in Psychology, 10.* doi:10.3389/fpsyg.2019.00467

Kowalski, R. M. (2001). *Behaving badly: Aversive behaviors in interpersonal relationships.* Washington, DC: American Psychological Association. https://doi.org/10.1037/10365-000

Meffert, H., Gazzola, V., den Boer, J. A., Bartels, A. A. J., & Keysers, C. (2013). Reduced spontaneous but relatively normal deliberate vicarious representations in psychopathy. *Brain, 136*(8), 2550–2562. doi:10.1093/brain/awt190

Neff, K. (2003). Self-compassion: An alternative conceptualization of a healthy attitude toward oneself. *Self and Identity, 2*(2), 85–101. doi:10.1080/15298860309032

Nummenmaa, L, Hirvonen, J, Parkkola, R, & Hietanen, J. K. (2008). Is emotional contagion special? An fMRI study on neural systems for affective and cognitive empathy. *Neuroimage, 43*, 571–80. doi:10.1016/j.neuroimage.2008.08.014

Paulhus, D. L., & Williams, K. M. (2002). The Dark Triad of personality: Narcissism, machiavellianism and psychopathy. *Journal of Research in Personality, 36*(6), 556–563. https://doi.org/10.1016/S0092-6566(02)00505-6

Schacter, D., Addis, D., & Buckner, R. (2007). Remembering the past to imagine the future: the prospective brain. *Nature Reviews Neuroscience 8*, 657–661. https://doi.org/10.1038/nrn2213

Shamay-Tsoory, S. G. (2011). The neural bases for empathy. *The Neuroscientist, 17*(1), 18–24. doi:10.1177/1073858410379268

Steinberg, D. (2010). Altruism in medicine: Its definition, nature, and dilemmas. *Cambridge Quarterly of Healthcare Ethics, 19*(02), 249. doi:10.1017/s0963180109990521

Tulving, E. (1985). "Memory and Consciousness". *Canadian Psychology, 26,* 1–12. doi:10.1037/h0080017

SECTION III.

AFFECTIVE MENTALIZING

To Simulate and Project

Chapter 3.

Affective Communication

Borderline Personality Disorder

Affective communication is an important aspect of human interaction, connecting people with one another on a deeper level. Affective communication can also, however, damage a relationship if dealt with carelessly. Affective miscommunication can be a problem in any relationship, but it is especially compounded by a condition known as borderline personality disorder (BPD). In the *Diagnostic and Statistical Manual of Mental Disorders* (American Psychiatric Association, 2022), the main features of borderline personality disorder (also called "emotionally unstable personality disorder") are defined as:

1. A pervasive pattern of instability of interpersonal relationships, self-image, and affects.
2. Marked impulsivity beginning by early adulthood and present in a variety of contexts.

BPD typically includes an unstable or dysfunctional self-image and a distorted image of others, in combination with an insecure world view. People with BPD generally suffer from feelings of emptiness, boredom and great emotional reactivity. For instance, they regularly display inappropriate outbursts of rage, often triggered by their misperceptions of events. They have a persistent fear of abandonment and rejection, which elicits severe anxiety and depression. This extreme emotional reactivity often comes with recurring self-destructive behaviors, such as self-mutilation. The way BPD individuals perceive themselves and the world around them leads to a history of unstable relationships that can change dramatically from intense love and idealization to devaluation and intense hatred. Kreisman and Straus (1989) aptly illustrate this intrapersonal conflict in the title of their book on BPD: *I Hate You—Don't Leave Me.*

BPD is often comorbid with other mental illnesses. For example, it occurs alongside of schizophrenia, mood and anxiety disorders, and narcissistic and psychopathic personality traits. BPD is over-represented in the mental health care system, due to its concomitant self-harm, mood disturbance, or psychotic-like symptoms, and in penitentiary populations, where comorbidity with psychopathic traits is most common. Affect dysregulation, as characterized by narcissism and psychopathy, are closely associated with BPD, and therefore alexithymia is assumed to be related, as a neurobiological factor, to the development of BPD as well.

Neurobiological factors play a crucial role in the development of BPD. These factors have a strong hereditary component according to research related to temperament, personality traits, neurology and neurochemistry. Nature, however, is not the only factor that explains the ontological development of this personality disorder. When we look at nurture, studies increasingly show that BPD often finds its roots in early childhood development. Theories of this nonbiological component focus predominantly on attachment relationships that people develop with their caregivers during childhood. We previously touched on attachment theory in relation to affective mentalizing. Levy detailed in his 2005 article that "one of the most consistent findings from initial studies examining the relationship between adult attachment and BPD is the association between unresolved disorganized attachment and BPD diagnosis (citations omitted)." This relationship can be understood by examining the "internal working model" of a person suffering from BPD. To reiterate from chapter 1 of this section, Affective Mentalizing, the concept of an "internal working model" was developed by Bowlby (1973), who described it as a representational system built up from past experiences with caregivers. To illustrate, a person with a secure attachment style has an internal working model that consists of a positive self-image and a positive view of others, combined with an interdependent attitude toward relationships and a low attachment avoidance. By contrast, individuals with BPD have an internal working model that is disorganized due to the interplay of their biological makeup in combination with negative experiences they have experienced with their early childhood caregivers. This disorganized internal working model is reflected in their unstable or dysfunctional self-image and distorted image of others, accompanied by an insecure world view. A key feature of disorganized attachment style is described by Main and Solomon (1986) as applying conflicting attachment strategies expressed through approach and avoidance behavior toward others. People with BPD commonly experience fight, flight and freeze reactions in their interactions with others.

People with BPD, and people with a disorganized attachment style in general, have yet another deficiency in common: *under-developed mentalization abilities*. Fonagy and Luyten argue that mentalization deficiencies are at the core of BPD behavior. In their 2009 article they explain:

"The failure of mentalizing, in combination with profound disorganization of self-structure, may account for the core features of borderline personality functioning." In the same article, Fonagy and Luyten contend that "a therapeutic intervention that focuses on the patient's capacity to mentalize in the context of attachment relationships can be helpful in improving both behavioral and affective aspects of the condition."

In light of the foregoing, we see that people with BPD have shortcomings in both the sending and the receiving of affective messages. They lack the ability to express their affective mental states appropriately in line with situational demands, and they often misread the affective messages of others. People who suffer from BPD comprise a population that represents extreme deficiencies in mentalization and affective communication. Milder mentalization and affective communication shortcomings are, however, also common in members of the general population.

Affective communication can be described as the affective information exchanges that guide our thinking and behavior. These information exchanges entail the encoding and decoding of affective messages. In her book entitled "*Communicating Emotions*," Planalp (1999) explains that our conversational goals are always accompanied by affects (emotions, moods and feelings). We get excited about a topic, we feel fear if our identity is threatened, we sense confusion if we can't follow what another person is saying. She describes three objectives that people typically pursue simultaneously in conversation:

1. Accomplishing a task (or achieving an instrumental goal)
2. Presenting oneself in a certain way
3. Managing social relationships

Our affects fluctuate depending on the level of importance we allocate to each of these goals. The more meaning we attach to a goal, the more affectively engaged we are with it. Generally, we attribute affects primarily to the content of the conversation. In truth, however, Planalp explains that affects are often elicited by the "relational meaning" that accompanies the conversation. To illustrate the importance of relational meaning, when a mother says *"Don't worry, mommy is here for you"* to her thirty-year-old son, information about how she views her relationship with her son is revealed in the way she refers to herself. When the mother's remark irritates her son, it is most likely the relational meaning that he finds annoying, not the fact that he does not need to worry, or that his mother wants to help him. Planalp also points out that the "coordination between partners in conversations occurs at many levels, and they are all grounds for emotions." Coordination covers conversational aspects such as sharing the same concern, agreeing on the topic of the conversation, taking turns during conversation and repairing misunderstandings. When our conversational objectives are not met, or our conversation goes off course, we tend to react emotionally. Most of the time, we reveal these emotions in our behavior, which elicits counter reactions from our conversational partner, often due to emotional or behavioral contagion, and outside of our conscious awareness. At such times, although we do communicate affective information, *we do not necessarily explain how we feel, what we feel, or why we feel it.*

Affective communication is a complex endeavor, not only because feelings can be triggered by a variety of factors, but also because different people do not necessarily react to the same factors in the same ways. The affects triggered in different individuals may vary in character or intensity based on differences in the expectations they have about a conversation, their self-image or their image of others, or the goals they want to reach through their interactions with others. Unexpected affective responses from others should alert people to the fact that an adjustment of their expectations or goals may be warranted. Affects prepare us to plan our behavior and motivate us to take action. Preparation may involve a conscious effort on our part, but it can also occur subconsciously. In addition, preparation can take place on the fly during a conversation, but it can also occur in advance of a conversation based upon affective forecasting. The preparations we make frequently find their basis in past experiences, tracing back as far as childhood. Such preparations, however, often cause us to disconnect from the current situation. Affective mentalizing plays a pivotal role in affective communication, enabling us to associate the affective changes that we detect in ourselves and others with their root causes. Affective mentalizing provides us with the opportunity to promptly address negative affective responses in real-time, keeping conversations and relationships on track. Similarly, the detection of positive affective changes in ourselves and others can serve as an indication that our communications are improving, and our relationships are becoming healthier.

Affective communication is an essential social competency. It enables us to establish a common emotional basis from which to work, and to reconnect with others if negative feelings begin to cloud our thinking or jeopardize our relationships. Moreover, it is critical to strengthening our connections with others through the sharing of positive and negative feelings and the deepening of mutual understanding. Affective communication is closely related to, but distinct from, empathy and compassion. While empathy and compassion have a clear recipient, affective communication involves a back-and-forth exchange of affective information *between people* in order to take, gain and shape one another's affective perspectives. In addition, while empathy and compassion are generally directed toward alleviating discomfort, affective communication includes the sharing of both *positive* and *negative* affects. Positive feelings and emotions such as appreciation, gratitude and delight are equally important to share, as they build and strengthen affectionate bonds. Appropriate affective information sharing helps us to reach our goals, to maintain a positive view of others and ourselves, to establish and deepen our connections, and to focus our mentalization efforts. Poor affective communication, on the other hand, generates fight, flight, or freeze reactions, especially when emotions run high, and conversations go off track.

Many people believe that communicating affectively is equivalent to clarifying one's feelings. In truth, however, affective communication can take place on two levels:

- First, we can communicate *affectively* through nonverbal behavioral displays, such as smiling, frowning, varying intonation, etc. This helps to *emphasize the affective component* of the verbal message we are sending (urgency, seriousness, etc.), but may still leave the observer in the dark about the meaning or underlying cause of our affective mental state.
- Second, we can communicate *affect* through verbal descriptions that *clarify the meaning or underlying cause of our affective mental states*. This "affective explaining" which is largely done through affective self-disclosure, will be discussed in greater detail in the next chapter.

There are two reasons that comprehensive affective communication requires the marrying of nonverbal affective displays with complementary verbal affective expressions:

- First, it requires us to align our verbal and nonverbal affective behavior to avoid incoherence and ambiguity in our affective communication.
- Second, it requires the ability to gather and interpret all relevant verbal and nonverbal affective information and to process that information into a coherent picture.

Nonverbal behavior adds meaning to verbal expression. It is critical to helping others understand how a message should be taken (literally, sarcastically, jokingly, etc.). Conversely, *verbal expression is critical to explain what feelings mean, to disclose feelings that are difficult to express using only nonverbal behavior, and to correct mistaken impressions.* Affective communication is comprised of three integrated and dynamic elements: affective explaining of experiences, affective message sending, and affective message receiving. We will continue with an examination of the first element: "affective explaining."

Affective Explaining

In order to explain our affective experiences and mental states to others, we need to understand the roles that verbal and nonverbal behavior play in communicating affect. In the book "*Nonverbal Communication*" by Burgoon et al. (2010), the authors explain that verbal expressions and nonverbal displays can work in different ways to get affective messages across. Let us first review how verbal behavior differs from nonverbal behavior:

- A first difference is that we use *multiple channels* when we communicate nonverbally, while we use a *single channel* (words) when we communicate verbally. Nonverbal displays enable us to communicate multiple messages at the same time. Although verbal expressions can have a double meaning, we are always limited to the single medium of words.
- A second difference is that verbal communication is *distinct* (linear) while nonverbal communication is *continuous* (fluid and context dependent). By distinct, we mean that messages have a clear beginning and end, and are expressed in a sequential fashion. Thus, while we can stop communicating verbally (at least most of us can), we never stop communicating nonverbally.
- A third difference is that we use verbal communication *consciously* while we generally communicate nonverbally on a *nonconscious* level.
- A fourth difference is that verbal communication is *dependent on the understanding of the meaning of words,* whereas some nonverbal communication is, generally speaking, *universally recognized*.
- A fifth and final difference is that *nonverbal behavior* is generally *harder to convey over certain media* than verbal communication. For instance, when we communicate via email, most nonverbal communication channels are blocked from the receiver. Because of this limitation, the affective undertone of written messages is often more dependent upon the reader's frame of mind than on the

intended impression of the writer. Emoticons have been introduced to bridge the affective nonverbal communication gap to a certain extent.

Making effective use of verbal and nonverbal communication is dependent upon an understanding of *how* and *when* to use the right communication channel. To illustrate, Burgoon et al. (2010) note that when we communicate affective mental states through nonverbal behavior, we *directly* impact the senses of others. Due to the influences of mimicry and affective contagion, we can invoke more rapid, automatic and affective reactions in others than we can with words. Burgoon et al. further explain that "verbal descriptions require an intermediate cognitive translation step before the individual can respond." Another required competence for effectual communication is the ability to understand what information we can share and with whom. Affective explaining, therefore, also relies upon our capacity for affective self-disclosure, as guided by well-developed sociocultural understanding.

"Self-disclosure" is, generally speaking, the act of communication by which people reveal personal or private information about themselves. The information can be descriptive or evaluative, and can include the disclosure of a wide range of mental states such as beliefs, intentions, preferences and dislikes. "Affective self-disclosure" focuses on the disclosure of affective mental states. According to social penetration theory, formulated by Altman and Taylor (1973), there are two dimensions to self-disclosure: breadth and depth. "Breadth" refers to the range of private and personal information that is revealed. "Depth" refers to increasingly sensitive, painful, or unusual information that is shared. People are generally more comfortable first expanding the breadth of information about themselves, such as various aspects of their affective experiences, before delving into more sensitive, painful, or unusual affects. Both dimensions are crucial to connecting with others on a deeper level and gaining a comprehensive perspective of affective mental states. Affective self-disclosure is most effective when the sender and receiver share a mutual state of mind that it is acceptable or appropriate to express feelings. There are times, however, when we have to explain our affective experiences to someone who is not necessarily receptive to hearing them. Such a situation requires a well-developed understanding of how to apply affective communication skills in light of the receiver's temperament, personality traits, sociocultural background, etc. To conclude, the process of affective self-disclosure needs to be managed well in order to assure that we are sharing our personal and private information with the right people, in the right way, and at the appropriate time and place.

Thus, well-developed affective explanation skills must include an understanding of:

- How to use our verbal and nonverbal communication skills effectively.
- How to explain affective experiences appropriately considering the context.
- The types of affective information that can be shared.
- The appropriate breadth and depth of the affective self-disclosure.
- When, and with whom, affective self-disclosure is appropriate.

When we affectively explain ourselves to others, we have to keep in mind that people are not mind readers in a magical or mystical sense. We need to assist others in reading our minds through acts of self-disclosure and through effective use of verbal and nonverbal behavior. Affective explaining is a competency that is useful beyond our own self-disclosures. We can also employ affective explaining skills to help others explain their affective experiences when they struggle with their own emotional self-disclosure. This is one of the key competencies of clinical psychologists. While affective explaining provides us with a way to help ourselves and others understand emotional experiences, it does not necessarily include targeted messaging designed to change the listener's perspective or behavior, as is the case with affective message sending. Let us explore what sending affective messages entails.

Sending Affective Messages

While affective explaining focuses on sharing emotional experiences with others, for instance, seeking advice from a psychotherapist, affective message sending focuses on how we relate our affective messages to others, not just to explain how we feel, but:

- to have people see the situation from our point of view, and
- to elicit a behavioral change in others.

This does not mean, however, that the aim of affective message sending is to convince others that our perspective is more valid than theirs. We merely ask them to momentarily set aside their own perspective, and perceive a situation as we do, or in other words, *to employ perspective shifting*. This helps others understand what is important to us and why we behave the way we do. Critical to sending affective messages, as with messages in general, is that they be as clear and concise as possible.

Linguist Paul Grice (1975) proposed the following communication guidelines, known as "Grice's maxims of conversation:"

- The maxim of "**quantity**," providing only as much information as is needed to inform.
- The maxim of "**quality**," providing only truthful information that is supported by evidence.
- The maxim of "**relation**," providing information that is relevant and pertinent to the discussion.
- The maxim of "**manner**," providing information in as clear, brief and orderly a fashion as possible to avoid obscurity and ambiguity.

Messages that are inconsistent or ambiguous can create miscommunication and misunderstanding. We often see this result when we are conflicted about something. For instance, when a father needs to discipline his misbehaving child, but at the same time finds what the child does to be amusing, he may address the behavior of the child in a clear and serious way while his facial expressions reveal his true feelings. These inconsistent or ambiguous messages are often also displayed in mixed-motive situations involving goals that are partially in consonance and partially in conflict, such as maintaining a good relationship with others while at the same time asking for more personal space. As with affective explaining, we need to align our verbal and nonverbal communication so that our message is coherent. We also need to choose the best way to explain what we feel and why we feel the way we do. Additionally, we need to communicate appropriately and clearly what the goal of our affective messages is, and what we expect from others in terms of behavioral changes.

Previously, we pointed out that in our interactions with others, affect is always running in the background. Even when our interactions with others are going smoothly, it is worthwhile to consciously monitor how all of the other participants are feeling (i.e., to employ affective mentalizing). Most of us, however, consider our own emotions (or those of others) only after they become salient, instead of monitoring them as a matter of course. When we fail to monitor affect during our interactions with others, emotional reactions often take us by surprise, and our resulting physiological reactions can intensify our feelings. The longer we wait to address the affective crescendo, the harder it becomes to stay focused on the conversation and on our conversational partner. Moreover, the delay undermines our ability to send or receive affective messages in a measured way. Notwithstanding the pressure we may feel to immediately tell another person how we feel under such circumstances, there are many good reasons to pause and consider the consequences before sending any "emotionally loaded" affective messages. Taking time in advance to consider the impact of affective messages goes a long way toward maintaining healthy relationships.

Preparing to send affective messages requires the integration of many different pieces of information, most of which are gathered through mentalization. As part of this preparation, we need to consider:

- ourselves as the sender,
- the recipient of the message, and
- the situational demands and contextual setting.

As senders of affective messages, we need to ask ourselves:

- *What am I truly feeling?*
- *Are my emotions influenced by fatigue or stress?*
- *What are the true causes of these feelings? Are they related to the behavior of the other person, the content of the conversation, or something in the environment? Am I just in a bad mood?*
- *How do influences such as personal goals or self-image factor into my affective mental state?*
- *What is my ultimate goal for sharing my feelings? Am I asking for a behavioral change? Am I asking for help? Am I looking for understanding and acceptance?*

The answers to these questions are derived through mentalizing about our own affects, desires, beliefs, etc. (i.e., intrapersonal mentalizing). When considering the recipient of our affective message we need to ask ourselves:

- *What do I know about this person? How is the person feeling? What does s/he want? What is my empathic forecast of the person's likely reaction to the message?*
- *Is the recipient stressed or fatigued? Is the person feeling the same emotions as I do? Do we differ in our experience of those emotions?*
- *Am I dealing with an empathetic person? Is this person susceptible to empathic distress or subject to some other affective impediment?*

The answers to these questions are provided through mentalizing about the affects, desires, beliefs, etc. of others (i.e., interpersonal mentalizing). When considering the situational demands and contextual setting (i.e., extrapersonal mentalizing), we need to ask ourselves:

- *Is it appropriate at this particular moment to send the affective message? If it is, what is the most effective way to do so?*
- *How revealing should I be in my affective self-disclosure? What are the cultural and contextual rules?*
- *What is the best medium to use for my affective message? Should I call the other person, deliver the message personally, or send the message in writing? If I send the message in writing, what is the appropriate written medium (e.g., text, email, formal letter, handwritten note)?*

Consideration of the aforementioned factors helps us to devise the best strategy for relating our affective messages. Moreover, we need to periodically assess the validity of our empathic forecasting, and adjust to unforeseen developments. Once again, mentalization underlies the entire process.

Appropriately crafted affective messages help others to see the situation from our point of view, and allow us to shape their perspectives. This is especially vital if we want other people to change their behavior in line with our own conversational goal. This aspect of affective communication is closely related to assertiveness. "Assertiveness" encompasses the capacity to express our concerns to others in a clear, concise and emphatic way so that they understand our perspective and respect our boundaries. We sometimes find it hard to communicate assertively about the way we feel. What are the reasons that we sometimes struggle to send affective messages in an assertive manner? We might think that the way we feel is unimportant, that the matter is not worthy of discussion, or that our feelings will go away on their own. We sometimes assume that others do not want to deal with our feelings or emotions. We may even see other people as our "enemies." Reluctance to inject feelings into a conversation can sometimes be attributable to sociocultural rules. Often, we simply do not know how to manage affective communication. This can be due to a failure to engage in the kind of self-oriented mentalization efforts that are required to gain a clear understanding of how we feel and what we want to accomplish with our affective messages. It can also be due to inadequate attention to the sort of other-oriented mentalization efforts that are required to gain a clear understanding of others, to know how we can best communicate with them, and to forecast their likely responses. Finally, it can be due to a failure to take situational factors into consideration.

Well-developed affective mentalizing competencies are required to strengthen affective message sending skills. Likewise, well-developed affective message sending skills help others to mentalize accurately about our own mental states, which in turn facilitates receiving the reaction from others that we are looking for. We now turn to the third component of affective communication: "receiving affective messages."

Receiving Affective Messages

We have seen that empathic, compassionate and affective communication behavior are all critical to accurate affective mentalizing. Likewise, affective mentalizing is heavily dependent on masterful affective message receiving skills and practices. Receiving affective messages requires us to shift perspectives; to consider the perspective of another while temporarily suspending our own. We can gain the perspectives of others only when our observations are unclouded by our own point of view. Additionally, it is important to keep in mind that affective messages are often sent by others with the objective of effecting a behavioral change in the receiver of the message. Thus, when properly received, the affective messages of others provide us with feedback in relation to our behavior toward the sender of the message, and in relation to our behavior in general. The receiving of affective messages, therefore, requires us to listen closely to the message, and to make sure we understand what the underlying stated or intended objective of the message is, including what the sender might be asking of us.

Finally, listening closely to the verbal accounts of others, while observing their nonverbal behavior, provides us with the opportunity to note discrepancies in their verbal and nonverbal behavior, inconsistencies about which even the sender might not be aware, but which can, nonetheless, reveal important information, such as internal conflicts or confusion with regard to important issues. We will now take a closer look at this last aspect of receiving affective messages: noting and decoding discrepancies.

Interestingly, discrepancies between subjective feelings and observable affective states are more evident at intermediate, as opposed to high levels of emotion. This means that although we tend to focus on salient or intense emotions, we need to engage our affective mentalizing abilities at the point where emotional behavior is less intense and often more subtle. Inconsistencies are a telltale sign that further consideration is warranted. Another important sign that there may be more going on than meets the eye is a disconnect between the affective message of the sender and the context or situation. When we sense that the message is unusually strong, weak, or inappropriate in relation to the situation and context, we need to probe into potential underlying causes for the apparent incongruity. Generally speaking, however, people are not particularly adept at using all of the available information channels to detect discrepancies in verbal and nonverbal behavior and/or situational incoherencies. To illustrate this point, social psychologists have studied whether we rely more heavily on verbal or nonverbal channels in making mental state inferences. Burgoon et al. (2010) proposed the following takeaways from available research:

- On average, adults rely more on nonverbal cues than on verbal cues to determine social meaning. Estimates in studies suggest that about 65% of the meaning in social context is conveyed nonverbally.
- Nonverbal cues prevail over verbal cues when: judging leadership and credibility; judging interpersonal styles; completing comprehension and behavioral tasks; answering interpretive questions; and distinguishing true attitudes, feelings and ideas from inconsistent expressions.

- Children rely more on verbal cues than adults do.
- Adults rely more on nonverbal cues when verbal and nonverbal channels conflict than when these channels are congruent.
- Communication channel reliance depends on the communication function at stake. Verbal content is more important for factual, cognitive, abstract and persuasive interpretations. Nonverbal content is more important for judging emotional and attitudinal expressions, relational communication and impression formation.
- When the content from different channels is congruent, the meanings of the cues tend to be averaged together equally; when content is incongruent, there is greater variability in how information is integrated.
- People have individual biases in their channel preference. Some people consistently rely on certain nonverbal channels, others rely more on verbal content, and still others adjust their preference for channels depending on the situation. People may rely on the channels they are best able to use and read depending on their particular skills.

Nonverbal communication adds even more complexity, as it is expressed through multiple channels, which often operate in parallel. As is the case with verbal and nonverbal communication, conflicts can occur between different nonverbal communication channels. Burgoon et al. explain further that we tend to have a primacy of visual cues. We rely heavily on visual cues:

- When mixed messages involve the face rather than the body.
- When decoding emotions related to positivity (agreeableness, gratitude, kindness).
- When the discrepancy between the visual and auditory codes is not large.

When it comes to decoding emotional information, visual cues are more semantically distinctive and are more efficient transmitters, providing more units of meaning per time unit. Humans may attend deliberately to the visual channel because, unlike auditory cues, it is not automatically alerting. This deliberate attention reduces the input from auditory cues, giving visual cues more impact. Encoders have greater control over their facial expressions, thereby providing decoders with more intentional information. Additionally, people may rely more on visual cues than on auditory cues because they can quickly scan someone's face and then concentrate on the most revealing facial cues, whereas with auditory cues, decoders must process the cues sequentially, and only fleetingly.

Thus, due to the greater amount of emotional information contained in the visual channel, the lower alerting capacity of visual cues, the greater intentionality potential and the longer duration of facial cues, people are believed to rely more on visual cues than on auditory cues when decoding mixed channel messages. There are notable exceptions to these conclusions. For instance, "body and vocalic cues become more important when receivers are decoding dominance, assertiveness, and anxiety" (Burgoon et al. 2010) (citing Scherer, Scherer, Hall, & Rosenthal, 1977; Zuckerman, Amidon, Bishop, & Pomerantz, 1982). Interestingly, many people assume that deception detection is best accomplished through visual cues. In fact, however, vocal tone is an equally powerful indicator of mental states, including deceptive intent. In addition, it is harder for people to consciously control their vocal tones than their facial expressions.

Receiving affective messages is not always an easy task. People are often uncertain about how to process "strong" affective messages from others. They can easily fall prey to affective contagion, displaying the same emotion (anger in response to anger) or a complementary emotion (fear in response to anger). Coping with assertiveness presents its own challenges. For instance, when we are on the receiving end of an assertive message, we might misinterpret the sender of the message as being aggressive or arrogant. This misinterpretation can give rise to negative emotions and increase feelings of stress, both of which tend to hinder mentalizing.

Whenever we are on the receiving end of an affective message it is important to keep in mind that people often send affective messages without even being aware of the fact that they are doing so. The best way to avoid misunderstandings in these circumstances is to invite the other person to self-disclose. In relation to receiving affective messages appropriately, we should focus not only on communications of negative emotions, but also on the communication of positive emotional messages. When listening to another person's affective self-disclosure, we need to distinguish between:

- The meaning of the sender's verbal and nonverbal behavior.
- The verbal content and tone of the sender's message.
- The meaning of the content to all parties concerned.
- The relational meaning to each of the parties.
- Our own goals in soliciting the disclosure and the goals that the sender is trying to achieve with the disclosure.

Content includes both the subject matter that is being discussed and the nature of the words being used during the disclosure. The relational level carries verbal and nonverbal information about the relationship between sender and receiver. It is often at the relational level that things become personal, and interactions become emotionally charged. We will now take a closer look at the interrelationship between affective mentalizing and affective communication.

The Interrelationship Between Affective Mentalizing and Affective Communication

A final challenge to affective communication remains: the factor of time. Given enough time, we are generally able to deliberate about the best way to communicate our affective experiences. Often, however, we do not have (or fail to take) the necessary time. Affective mentalizing provides a practical solution to this problem. Through the application of affective mentalizing we are able to train ourselves to be mindful of the affective mental states that underlie our interactions from the moment we first engage with others. This helps us to set a baseline for our own affective mental states and for the affective mental states of others. This baseline is critical to detecting changes in affective mental states before they distract us from the objective of the interaction.

As we have seen, affective mentalizing involves the conscious monitoring and regulation of fluctuations in the affective mental states of ourselves and others. We detect these fluctuations through primary sensory information, nonverbal behavior and verbal accounts. Affective mentalizing enables us to get to know ourselves and others better. Additionally, it is instrumental to assuring that we address uncomfortable feelings and acknowledge positive feelings (both our own and those of others) in a timely and context-relevant fashion. Initially, this monitoring might sound unduly effortful. Through training and practice, however, the process becomes more natural. One way to gauge our affective mentalizing and communication competencies is to consciously monitor the "fluidity" of our interactions with others. So how can we tell if our interactions are fluid?

Detecting Signs of Fight, Flight or Freeze Mental States

We can recognize fluidity in a conversation when the interaction is perceived as comfortable, effortless and frictionless. This quality of information exchange is often described as flow. "Conversational flow" establishes a strong sense of connection among all of the parties to a conversation. The flow of conversation usually entails an affective component. All of the parties should feel welcome to express their feelings and emotions as they arise. Good flow is evident from the tacit acknowledgement (verbal or nonverbal) *"I'm OK, you're OK."* Good flow helps us to establish a win-win mindset in our interactions with others. A conversation with good flow focuses on the cooperative rather than the competitive nature of the exchange, and reduces the urge of participants to act defensively or out of provocation. Good interactional flow promotes good mentalization at all levels. Let us take a look at the signs that interactional flow is lacking.

The following three reactive states reveal conversation patterns that have the potential to restrict or undermine mentalization, or to take it offline altogether. When conversations are not in flow, we often detect mental states of competition, resignation, or rigidness through fight, flight, or freeze reactions. Communication in a "fight" state is indicated, *inter alia,* by competition regarding the content or the process of the conversation, by emphasis on the status of the participants, or by a perceived threat to identities and goals. A fight state creates a win-lose mindset. Communication in a "flight" state is marked by abdication of the opportunity for self-expression and surrender of space to negotiate the content, process or outcome of the interaction, and/or relinquishment of personal status. In a flight state, we tend to hasten the conclusion of the interaction. The outcome that such a reaction yields is a lose-win mindset. Bilateral communication in a "freeze" state ceases altogether. A freeze state signifies a confrontation between participants in which no one can proceed or retreat without being exposed to the threat of being perceived as the "loser." It is sometimes referred to as a "Mexican standoff." Participants in a freeze state feel as though they need to maintain strategic tension. This tension often remains unresolved until some outside event or influence breaks the impasse. The outcome that a freeze reaction yields is a lose-lose mindset; nobody wins and everybody loses.

When we detect signs of fight, flight, or freeze mental states through affective mentalizing, we need to redirect our focus to improving affective communication. This redirection serves several goals. Most importantly, it serves to diffuse the intensity of emotions and feelings of stress through validation, to explain or understand moods (depression, irritation), and to become aware of contributing physical states (hunger, fatigue, pain), all of which can hinder the flow of our communication and our ability to mentalize. Redirection also promotes understanding of the underlying cause of these affective states, which in turn serves the goal of keeping relationships healthy and promoting objectives. In sum, affective communication is strengthened through well-developed affective mentalizing competencies, and affective mentalizing is reinforced by well-developed affective communication competencies.

Affect Regulation

Affective mentalizing serves yet another important purpose. Affective mentalizing promotes affect self- and other-regulation. Affect self-regulation is necessary to keep our own emotions in check during challenging or highly charged interactions. Affect regulation is such an integral part of our behavior that we do it largely on a subconscious level. Planalp (1999) explains that "we regulate emotions often unconsciously and automatically, having started regulating emotions early in life." We need to learn to employ affect regulation on a conscious level, and in a goal-directed manner. This is not always easy to do. Planalp, for instance, argues that "[p]eople seldom have the luxury to sit back and reflect on their emotions during conversations." According to Planalp, this is due to the fact that "[a]ttention fluctuates among the many different aspects of conversation – the content, the process, the other people involved, our own thoughts and our own feelings." We can and should apply sound affect regulation strategies in all aspects of our communications. For example:

- We can divert our attention away from or toward the cause of an emotion.
- We can change our appraisal of the situation.
- We can adjust our physical response.
- We can address the cause of the emotion.

- We can evaluate and choose the best behavioral response to what we see, think, feel, etc.

Not only can we regulate our own affective states, but we can also influence the affective states of others. Through the conscious employment of phenomena such as affective contagion, we are able to regulate the affective states of others, for instance, by toning down our own emotions, or by amplifying them, as appropriate. We can also influence the feelings of others to be more positive or negative. Our level of awareness of affective mental and physical states correlates positively with the opportunities that we perceive to control and regulate those affective states. This awareness is fostered and enhanced through affective intrapersonal mentalizing. We will now continue with an examination of the key advantages of good affective communication.

Affective Communication Skills: Advantages, Impediments and Avenues for Enhancement

ADVANTAGES

Good affective communication practices yield multiple benefits. From an intrapersonal perspective, *competent affective communication attracts affection and appreciation*. Good senders (or encoders) of affective messages tend to be well-adjusted and extroverted - communicating in a more expressive, engaging and coordinated fashion. They tend to have higher self-esteem and a higher level of emotional complexity, both of which enable them to understand themselves and others better. Their nonverbal behaviors are more flexible and well-suited to the situation, adding to the clarity and persuasiveness of their messages. They engage more readily in self-monitoring. Good receivers (or decoders) of affective messages - tend to be more sociable and better listeners, more self-effacing and less self-centered. They are good at role-playing and creating favorable impressions. They excel in mentalizing, which helps them to size up other people. Interestingly, good encoding skills do not necessarily translate into good decoding skills, and vice versa. Therefore, in order to become an adept affective communicator, we need to develop both good encoding skills and good decoding skills.

On an interpersonal level, studies show that *healthy affective communication enhances trust between people.* Appropriate affective self-disclosure, in particular, helps us to connect with others on a deeper level. Enhanced trust, in turn, enhances affective mentalizing. Moreover, our demonstrated ability to accurately identify and describe not only basic emotions, moods and feelings, but also blended and complex affective mental states, *helps others to see things from our perspective, and thus, to accurately mentalize about us,* which in turn significantly increases our ability to elicit desired responses and behavioral changes in others. Research indicates, for instance, that individuals who can articulate the nature and underlying causes of their anxieties are more likely to receive reassuring and compassionate reactions from others. Such individuals also use their affective communication skills to invite others to share their own affective messages in a clear and effective manner. In return, they are perceived as receptive and trustworthy friends.

On an extrapersonal level, skillful affective communication requires that we take contextual demands into account in deciding how and when to communicate affectively. *Well-crafted affective messages that take sociocultural and other situational factors into account are more easily understood and less likely to lead to social faux pas.* People with well-developed bilateral affective communication skills are well liked and respected within the larger community.

IMPEDIMENTS

Impediments to affective communication exist on three levels as well. On an intrapersonal level, for instance, *discomfort with emotional topics can cause us to avoid situations that might require us to share feelings with others.* This can cause us to become rigid in our communication and isolate ourselves from others. It can also impede us from gaining insight into our own affective mental states and learning about ourselves. Emotional discomfort can lead us to suppress our feelings, increasing the chances that we will react inappropriately in our dealings with others. Suppressed feelings can bias our perceptions and cause us to become irritated with others. For many people, sharing feelings does not come naturally; it has to be learned.

From an interpersonal perspective, *our affective communication often goes awry if the affective message is not sent or received completely.* This can be due to a lack of attention, inadequacies in the abilities or skills needed to encode or decode affective messages, or projection of our own mental states on others. In addition, *our reciprocal affective communications are impacted by the affective communication competencies of those with whom we communicate.* This can often elicit feelings of awkwardness or discomfort. Good affective communication can also be impeded by a *lack of connectedness or common ground.* This can be due, for instance, to sociocultural factors, lack of affinity, or a perceived disparity in status. Through the application of our basic mentalizing skills, we are able to readily pick up on disconnections that can make it difficult to discuss our feelings, resonate with others and achieve a mutual understanding.

On an extrapersonal level, affective communication becomes increasingly difficult in complex and unstable social environments. People may withhold, or conversely, inappropriately share, their affective mental states because they are not sufficiently familiar with applicable sociocultural rules, or because those rules restrict the freedom to express or respond to affective states. Unfamiliarity with sociocultural rules can lead to embarrassing social faux pas. Other situational demands can constrain our ability to communicate in the optimal manner. Various electronic communication media, for instance text message, email, teleconferencing, etc., can make communicating about sensitive topics a very challenging and frustrating endeavor. We will now examine opportunities that exist for enhancing our affective communication competencies.

AVENUES FOR ENHANCEMENT

Affective communication deals with the most sensitive aspects of our interpersonal interactions. Affective communication can go awry easily. Absent proper course correction of miscommunications, mentalizing is taken offline and relationships are left hanging in the balance. The following competencies are essential tools in the arsenal of a skillful affective communicator:

- Monitoring of affective nonverbal behavior (basic mentalizing) and affective verbal indicators for early detection of changes in affective mental states. The capacity to survey affective states and assess their influence is critically important to detecting fight, flight and freeze reactions in a timely manner, lowering stress levels, reducing negative emotions and repairing interactional flow.
- Affective message encoding, through the alignment of our own verbal and nonverbal communication to enhance message clarity and impact, which requires us:
    - To understand how verbal and nonverbal communication channels work together most effectively in light of the situation, our conversational counterparts and our conversational objectives. This involves communicating affectively through nonverbal behavioral displays, such as smiling, frowning, varying intonation, etc., and using verbal descriptions to clarify the meaning or underlying cause of affective mental states.
    - To understand what appropriate affective self-disclosure entails, and know when, where, how and with whom to share our affective experiences, taking into consideration our objectives as the sender, the intended recipient and the situational demands and contextual setting.
    - To have a good understanding of the impact of affect in relation to the objectives of the communication. The four primary objectives in our communications with others are:

to accomplish a task or achieve an instrumental goal, to present ourselves in a particular way, and to manage our social relationships. Each of these objectives can inject its own affective elements into a conversation. Moreover, the coordination aspects of conversational flow (topic, turn taking, etc.) can all give rise to their own affective considerations.

- To recognize affective communication impediments in others so that we can adjust our communication style and expectations accordingly.
- To promote affect self- and other-regulation through calming and reassuring verbal and nonverbal behavior during challenging or highly charged interactions, a skill essential to keeping affective states like negative emotions and stress in check, and keeping our mentalization faculties online. Alternatively, it may be more appropriate to elicit excitement and positive energy when others have a hard time connecting to a positive affective message that you share with them.

- Affective message decoding, through the assembly and interpretation of affective information to make accurate affective mental state inferences. This competency requires us to be able:
  - To coordinate all of our information gathering channels, both verbal and nonverbal (i.e., visual, audio).
  - To temporarily suspend our own affective perspective in deference to the affective perspectives of others (perspective shifting).
  - To detect discrepancies within and between affective verbal and nonverbal behavior and ask for clarifications to understand others to the best of our ability.
  - To react in an appropriate way to both negative and positive affective disclosures and messages from others.

As with any attempt to enhance our mentalizing competencies, we first need to establish a baseline through a self-assessment of the affective mentalizing competencies by which we detect changes in affective mental states that could lead to fight, flight, or freeze reactions. Finally, we need to assess the affective message encoding and decoding competencies that we use to facilitate accurate and comprehensive verbal and nonverbal affective social indicator sharing.

SECTION SUMMARY

As we conclude this final chapter of our section on affective mentalizing, we would like to summarize the various concepts that have been discussed elsewhere in this section. In the first chapter of this section, we discussed the importance of having a positive attitude toward affect, and a well-developed affective understanding, for accurate affective mentalizing. We examined how attitude toward affect is formed, and how this attitude influences our affective understanding of self and others. Additionally, we discussed how a deeply and broadly developed comprehension of emotions, feelings and moods increases our ability to engage in complex affective thinking. In the second chapter we explored the progression from affective contagion and affect indicator processing, through basic and affective mentalizing, to empathizing with others and acting compassionately. We examined the difference between two forms of empathy - affective empathy and cognitive empathy - and the influence of empathic distress on compassionate behavior. Furthermore, we discussed how empathizing and acting compassionately can be guided by affective mentalizing, and how the effectiveness of our empathetic and compassionate behavior can, in turn, inform the accuracy of our affective mentalizing inferences. In the current chapter we have examined affective communication, which encompasses the exchange of affective information between people, and we discussed the interrelationship between affective mentalizing and affective communication. In the next section, we are going to explore the highest level of mentalizing: "strategic mentalizing."

References

Altman, I., & Taylor, D. A. (1973). *Social penetration: The development of interpersonal relationships.* Holt, Rinehart, & Winston, New York, 459.

American Psychiatric Association (2022). *Personality Disorders. In Diagnostic and statistical manual of mental disorders* (DSM-5-TR). American Psychiatric Association Publishing.

Bowlby, J., (1973) *Attachment and Loss: Separation, Anxiety and Anger.* Basic Books, New York.

Burgoon, J. K., Guerrero, L. K., & Floyd, K. (2010). *Nonverbal communication.* Taylor & Francis.

Fonagy, P., & Luyten, P. (2009). A developmental, mentalization-based approach to the understanding and treatment of borderline personality disorder. *Development and Psychopathology, 21*(04), 1355. doi:10.1017/s0954579409990198

Grice, H. P. (1975). *Logic and conversation.* In P. Cole & J. J. Morgan (Eds.), *Syntax and Semantics 3: Speech Acts* (p. 41–58). New York, NY: Academic Press.

Kreisman, J. J., & Straus, H (1989). *I Hate You--Don't Leave Me.* New York: Avon Books.

Levy, K. N. (2005). The implications of attachment theory and research for understanding borderline personality disorder. *Development and Psychopathology, 17*(04). doi:10.1017/s0954579405050455

Main, M., & Solomon, J. (1986). *Discovery of an insecure-disorganized/disoriented attachment pattern.* In T. B. Brazelton & M. W. Yogman (Eds.), *Affective development in infancy* (p. 95–124). Ablex Publishing.

Planalp, S. (1999). *Communicating Emotion: Social, Moral, and Cultural Processes.* Cambridge University Press.

SECTION IV.

STRATEGIC MENTALIZING

To Reason and Evaluate

Chapter 1.

Motivation to Mentalize Strategically

Introduction to Strategic Mentalizing

Strategic mentalizing, the highest level of mentalization, involves reasoning about mental states on a more abstract level in order to make accurate theory of mind inferences. We start this section by reviewing where strategic mentalizing fits within the full scope of mentalization. We will then elaborate on what strategic mentalizing entails, and provide a brief description of the four constituent components of strategic mentalizing. Against this backdrop, we will introduce the topic of this chapter: the motivation to strategically mentalize.

A MULTI-COMPONENT ABILITY

As we have seen, mentalization is a multi-component ability. Although all components are heavily interrelated, we can distinguish three levels of mentalization:

- Basic mentalizing
- Affective mentalizing
- Strategic mentalizing

Strategic mentalizing is the highest and most cognitive level of mentalization. It enables us to look beyond observable signals and cues to form increasingly rational models of what is going on in the minds of others. It is on this strategic level that we are able to make theory of mind inferences. We refer to this level as "strategic mentalizing" because it involves two distinct strategic orientations and objectives: first, *to enhance affiliation and cooperation*; and second, *to distance from others and/or gain a competitive advantage*. Often, however, our motives for interacting with others are not exclusively directed to either enhancing cooperation or gaining competitive advantage. Many social interactions, such as negotiations, involve overlapping goals, so that both enhancing cooperation and gaining competitive advantage play a role. These "mixed-motive" situations require increasingly complex higher-order mentalization.

FOCUS ON EPISTEMIC MENTAL STATES

Strategic mentalizing focuses on the more epistemic (cognitive) mental states - desires, beliefs and knowledge. It is on this strategic level that *verbal* communication becomes a strong focal point, since we are not able to infer the more cognitive mental states through observation alone. Nonetheless, nonverbal communication still plays a pivotal role in our understanding of the minds of others, and therefore strategic mentalizing is informed by both basic and affective mentalizing. Strategic mentalizing enables us to move from common-sense or folk psychology to increasingly rational theory of mind inferences that are based on psychological and sociological understanding substantiated by empirical evidence. Strategic mentalizing provides us with the ability to test our common-sense inferences against alternative models of, or explanations for, human behavior. It is on this level of mentalization that we take all rational explanations for human behavior into account, even counterintuitive aspects that challenge our common-sense inferences. Studies repeatedly show that we often err in our assumptions about the mental states and behavior of others. This becomes evident when we look at the different ways our perceptions of others can be biased, which we will address later in this section.

THE KEY FEATURES

What are the key features of strategic mentalizing efforts? Strategic mentalizing is *cognitive, conscious,* and *explicit.* This level of mentalization is generally *offline,* and must either be triggered by external events, or consciously brought online. It is often *employed outside of the immediate interaction,* either to prepare for social encounters before they occur, or to evaluate such events after the fact. The information flow is *verbal, rational, strategic* and *specific to the individual.* The advantages of mentalizing on this level are that it is *complex, sophisticated* and *flexible,* which significantly enhances accuracy in complex situations. Furthermore, we have a *high level of control* over this level. The limitations of strategic mentalizing are that it is *slow, deliberative* and *relatively effortful.*

METACOGNITIVE PROCESSES

Though the three levels of mentalization are heavily intertwined, the concept of strategic mentalizing can be distinguished from basic and affective mentalizing by examining metacognitive processes. "Metacognitive processes" entail thinking about how people's thoughts come about. Strategic mentalizing components overlap with the components associated with metacognitive thinking. Basic and affective mentalizing primarily concern a *reflection* on mental states, to a large extent involving the mental state of affect, and the more elementary, observable indicators of intent. Basic mentalizing focuses on nonverbal behavior in taking the perspectives of others, while affective mentalizing primarily concerns the reflection on affective mental states through simulation or projection. To a large extent, basic and affective mentalizing are accomplished in an implicit and spontaneous fashion. By contrast, on the strategic mentalizing level, the processes are *explicit* and *relatively effortful*. "Explicit mentalizing" involves conscious reflection upon the motives and mental states of ourselves and others. In other words, we think about what we and others are feeling, desiring, believing and knowing, and consider how we and others arrived at these mental states. We use this social information to form complex mental state inferences in order to explain and predict behavior. This is the essence of the component of metacognitive thinking that overlaps with higher-level mentalization. We can never be absolutely sure, however, of what other people are thinking or feeling, and our own thoughts and feelings are often vague and unclear, as well. Strategic mentalizing is, therefore, best viewed as a form of "probabilistic reasoning" (problem-solving techniques based on the use of probability theory to indicate the uncertainty in knowledge when weighing evidence and inferring conclusions).

EIGHT THEORY OF MIND DIMENSIONS

Until recently, researchers have viewed strategic mentalizing as a unitary cognitive construct, rather than as a diverse set of distinct functions. Within the last two decades, however, neuroscientists have discovered that there are several dimensions of theory of mind reasoning, with each strategic mentalizing dimension having a different neurological underpinning. In our study of the available literature, we have identified eight different theory of mind dimensions that relate to strategic mentalizing:

1. "**Affective**" **theory of mind**. This involves the rational consideration of the possible influences that affects can have on the increasingly epistemic mental states of desire, belief and knowledge, and on the

more complex mental states of intention, attitude and motivation. Affective theory of mind is distinguishable from affective mentalizing. The distinction lies in the way we *process* affective information, and in the *purposes* for which we apply our understanding of affective states. When we process affect signals through simulation and projection in the course of interactions with others, in order to keep our mentalization efforts online and maintain healthy relationships, we are engaging in *affective mentalizing*. When we explicitly consider the possible influence affective states can have on the more epistemic mental states in our attempts to explain or predict behavior, we are engaging in *affective theory of mind reasoning*. Thus, whereas affective theory of mind relies on *cognitive reasoning* to infer mental states in order to explain past behavior or predict future behavior, affective mentalizing relies on *simulation* and *projection* to employ empathetic and compassionate behavior, and on the sharing of affective mental states in order to elicit reciprocal sharing by others, and to keep mentalization faculties online during emotionally charged situations.

2. "**Cognitive**" **theory of mind**. This involves reasoning about the increasingly epistemic mental states of desire, belief and knowledge, and the more complex mental states, in order to make predictions and come up with explanations of behavior.
3. "**Conative**" **theory of mind**. This involves reasoning about affective and cognitive mental states with the underlying intention of influencing the cognitive and affective mental states of others through purposeful communication, for instance, using ironic criticism or empathic praise.
4. "**Intrapersonal**" **theory of mind**. This involves reasoning about our own cognitive and affective mental states in order to gain insight into the reasons for our past behavior, or to predict our future behavior.
5. "**Interpersonal**" **theory of mind**. This involves reasoning about the cognitive and affective mental states of others with whom we have

direct interaction, in order to gain insight into the reasons for their past behavior or to predict their future behavior.

6. "**Extrapersonal**" **theory of mind**. This involves reasoning about the cognitive and affective mental states of larger groups of people outside of our personal interaction, in order to gain insight into the reasons for their past behavior, or to predict their future behavior. Additionally, it includes taking the situational context into account when reasoning about mental states.
7. "**Cooperative/affiliative**" **theory of mind**. This involves mental state reasoning oriented toward enhancing cooperation and affiliation with others.
8. "**Competitive/social distancing**" **theory of mind**. This involves mental state reasoning oriented at improving our competitive advantage over others or distancing ourselves from others.

The first two of these dimensions, affective and cognitive theory of mind, integrate information from both affective and cognitive mental states, assembled from different areas of the brain. The third dimension, conative theory of mind, uses the assembled mental state information to select communication strategies designed to purposefully influence others by recruiting other brain regions to make this possible. The following three dimensions, intra-, inter- and extrapersonal theory of mind, use different regions of the brain in concert with directional focus on the subject matter of our strategic mentalizing. The final two dimensions, cooperative/affiliative and competitive/social distancing theory of mind, indicate two distinct strategic directions that involve still other regions of the brain. Although a comprehensive explanation of the precise brain regions is beyond the scope of this chapter, our intent here is to illustrate the complexity of theory of mind reasoning.

Strategic mentalizing takes on a critical role when communication is ambiguous, complex and uncertain, and/or when the consequences of misinterpretation are potentially dire. The more proficient we are at strategic mentalizing, the less susceptible we are to misunderstandings and faulty predictions. In a sense, we all are "teleologists," in that we naturally attempt to explain behavior as a function of its end, purpose, or objective. This is not done simply by reasoning about what another person should have done or ought to do, or by conjuring up random explanations and predictions. Our reasoning needs to be based on mental states, goals, temperament, personality, context and other behavioral influences. For instance, when one person is more fully informed than another person, both individuals can reach very different decisions. We also need to keep in mind that people sometimes simply act irrationally. Strategic mentalizing relies upon reasoning, rather than simulation or self-projection, to supply an understanding of mental states.

DIFFERENT ORDERS OF THEORY OF MIND ATTRIBUTION

The *cognitive* theory of mind dimension of strategic mentalizing is associated with several different "orders" of theory of mind attribution. These mental state attributions may relate to different epistemic mental states such as desire, belief, or knowledge. Examples of theory of mind attributions can be found in literature such as crime novels or fairy tales. The first three orders of cognitive theory of mind attribution of mental states are described below:

- "**Zeroth-order**" **cognitive theory of mind attribution** (e.g., "I think it is raining outside," or "I believe I am good at this game"), involves *non*social reasoning, which does not take the mental states of others into account.
- "**First-order**" **cognitive theory of mind attribution**, involves recursive evaluation of the zeroth level (e.g., "I think that you think it is raining outside," or "I think she knows the rules of the game better than I do"), which allows us to reason about the mental states of others.
- "**Second-order**" **cognitive theory of mind attribution**, adds a further evaluation to consideration of the minds of others (e.g., "I think that you think that she thinks it is raining," or "I think that she thinks that he thinks he knows the rules of the game better than she

does"). It involves predicting what one person thinks about another person's mental state.

With each addition of a new perspective from another person to the chain of perspectives, we create a higher-order theory of mind attribution. Thus, the complexity of attribution increases with each new order. Adults are able to make fourth-order cognitive theory of mind attributions reasonably well. Above the fourth level, however, the accuracy rate falls off dramatically. Higher-order theory of mind reasoning is essential for strategic mentalizing, as it is required for navigation of complex social situations involving multiple people, for instance, socially intricate work environments or interactions involving strategic competition. Interestingly, De Weerd et al. explain in their 2018 article:

> The human ability to make use of higher-order theory of mind is especially apparent in story comprehension tasks. ... [E]xperimental evidence shows that people have more difficulty applying their theory of mind abilities in strategic games. In these settings, individuals are typically found to reason at low orders of theory of mind and are slow to adjust their level of theory of mind reasoning to more sophisticated opponents (citation omitted). However, some empirical research suggests that the use of theory of mind by participants can be facilitated by context (citations omitted), setting (citation omitted), and training (citations omitted).

THEORY OF MIND IS NOT EQUAL TO SOCIAL INTELLIGENCE

When we engage in strategic behavior to form alliances, or to compete with others, we act in a socially intelligent way. This does not, however, necessarily mean that we are making theory of mind inferences. In other words, *we should not confuse social intelligence with theory of mind.* Theory of mind requires that we take the *mental states* of others into consideration. In his 1999 article on the evolution of theory of mind, Baron-Cohen cited eight behaviors that depend on theory of mind reasoning:

1. Intentionally communicating with others
2. Repairing failed communication with others
3. Teaching others
4. Intentionally persuading others
5. Intentionally deceiving others
6. Building shared plans and goals
7. Intentionally sharing a focus or topic of attention
8. Pretending

Social intelligence can take us a long way, especially within a society with which we are familiar, or with likeminded people. Even in these circumstances, however, communication can go awry. In order to reach the communication goals listed by Baron-Cohen, we need to form "metarepresentations" of the mental states of others, and contrast those metarepresentations with our own mental states. For instance, when a builder communicates with a prospective customer in connection with a renovation plan, the builder cannot rely solely on socially intelligent (i.e., professional) behavior. The builder also needs to gain an understanding of the prospect's concepts for the renovations, appreciation of the structural implications, the investment required, etc. The builder and the prospect need to contrast and connect their mental states to make sure that their desires and expectations are aligned. Let us explore the constituent elements of strategic mentalizing.

FOUR COMPONENTS OF STRATEGIC MENTALIZING

We have divided strategic mentalizing into four components. Each component is the subject of a separate chapter. The current chapter, *Motivation to Mentalize Strategically,* relates to our motivation to employ strategic mentalizing efforts. Here we discuss how intrapersonal, interpersonal and extrapersonal factors influence our motivation to strategically mentalize about others.

In the second chapter, *Content Extraction,* we focus on the type of information we look for when we strategically mentalize. On the strategic mentalizing level, we need to gather signals and cues that reveal all possible mental states (including affective states), but especially the increasingly epistemic mental states of desire, belief and knowledge, to make comprehensive theory of mind inferences. We do this by extracting relevant and probative information from verbal accounts, and combining and contrasting this information with nonverbal behavior.

In the third chapter, *Perspective Gaining and Shifting*, we examine how we use strategic mentalizing competencies to gain insight into the perspectives of others, and to contrast these perspectives with our own. We also examine the concept of attributional complexity, which is pivotal to determining the most probable predictions or explanations of behavior.

In the fourth chapter, *Perspective Shaping*, we discuss how strategic mentalizing can strengthen our power to influence others, and to resist the unwanted influence of others. We now continue with an examination of the first component, our motivation to mentalize strategically. To set the stage we will look at how a famous film director used strategic mentalizing masterfully to create a mental state of suspense.

The Master of Suspense

"The Master of Suspense," Sir Alfred Joseph Hitchcock, is well known for his unmatched ability to motivate audiences to mentalize about his movie characters. As many of us know, Hitchcock was a British film director and producer, directing over 50 feature films over six decades. He is recognized as one of the greatest minds in the history of cinema. Well-known examples of his work include Psycho, Vertigo and The Birds. Hitchcock earned his reputation as the Master of Suspense through his talent for keeping audience members on the edge of their seats, drawing movie-goers into the psychological states of his characters. His audiences find themselves glued to the screen, trying to predict what is going to happen next. How did Hitchcock succeed in making the audience mentalize about his characters with such strong attentional focus? He understood exactly how to draw his audience into the minds of the characters by engaging the viewers' mentalization skills. Hitchcock's cinematic style included using camera movement to mimic a person's gaze, and framing shots so as to maximize the visibility of the facial expressions of anxiety and fear. His emphasis on actors' emotional expressions and glances kept viewers spellbound. As Hitchcock described it himself, "[t]here is no terror in the bang, only in the anticipation of it." Hitchcock believed that information and suspense went hand in hand. He showed the audience what the character couldn't see. He knew that a good way to create suspense was to let his audience in on something the protagonist did not know. Hitchcock made his audience juggle two perspectives, that of the character and that of the viewer. He made the audience contemplate what the character would do if he had all of the information available to the viewer, and what the character would be likely to do without it. Thus, Hitchcock audiences were left trying to predict the future based upon the knowledge state of the character.

One of the other tactics that Hitchcock employed to create suspense was his selection of his leading ladies. They had the capacity to mesmerize the audience in unconventional and unpredictable ways. Hitchcock recognized that the looming feelings of terror and suspense increased the audience's motivation to mentalize. Hitchcock fans entered the movie theater with an expectation of suspense, a form of affective forecasting. The inclination to strategically mentalize was, therefore, already heightened even before the characters were projected on the silver screen. We will now continue with a discussion of the core principles of this chapter.

As previously mentioned, basic and affective mentalizing rely less on cognitive resources and motivation than does strategic mentalizing. This comes with a tradeoff, however, as basic and affective mentalizing have more limited utility when it comes to explaining complex interactions or predicting behavior. Theory of mind inferences are rarely straightforward, and often rely heavily on the motivation of the mentalizer.

Motivational Factors for Strategic Mentalizing

Factors that mediate the transition from simple detection and sharing of mental states to strategic mentalizing include: the person with whom we are interacting, the salience, importance and ambiguity of a situation, the time and effort (we have or are willing to apply), and the strength of our motivation to understand the intentions of others.

Our motivation to mentalize about others is often influenced by affective mental states, such as irritation or confusion, related to the actions of others, or by feelings of uncertainty in highly ambiguous situations. Similarly, our affective disposition can increase or decrease our motivation to mentalize. To illustrate, people who suffer from social anxiety have a strong desire to know what people around them are thinking (especially about them), while individuals who suffer from depression are less likely to effortfully mentalize about others. Some people are simply more naturally inclined to engage in the efforts required for theory of mind analysis, while other more transient state of mind factors can also have a significant impact on the motivation to strategically mentalize. Strategic mentalizing is, therefore, both trait and state driven, as is the case with basic and affective mentalizing.

Our motivation to engage in strategic mentalizing is especially strong when we meet new people, as we want to ascertain whether or not they are trustworthy. We generally evaluate others on different dimensions of "trust." Two core dimensions of trust upon which we gauge others are:

1. **"Integrity"** (i.e., honesty, loyalty, responsibility, compassion, respect, fairness and citizenship).
2. **"Competence"** (i.e., technical skills, experience, reliability and power).

Put simply, we try to answer two questions:

1. *Do I want to affiliate with this person?*
2. *Will this person add value to the affiliation?*

Interestingly, Fiske et al. (2002) found in their study that while someone's *competence* is highly valued, it is evaluated only after *trust* in their level of integrity has been established. Initial judgments of trustworthiness are generally achieved through our *lower* mentalization levels. The evaluation of these judgements is, however, largely based on strategic mentalizing, which is vital to making beneficial affiliation decisions. Prevost et al., for instance, found in their 2015 study that judging the trustworthiness of strangers is associated with theory of mind skills. They studied both healthy individuals and individuals with paranoid personality disorder. These researchers concluded that,

> paranoid patients' better ability to read others' minds was associated with judging others as more trustworthy, while the reverse was found in the healthy participants (better mindreading was associated with judging others as less trustworthy), suggesting a non-linear relationship between trust in others and being able to read their intentions.

Our motivation to mentalize varies depending on who the subject of our attention is. The nature of our interpersonal relationship with a person affects our motivation to mentalize about that person. For instance, we mentalize more readily about people whom we view as having a higher status than we do. Additionally, we tend to generate more nuanced and detailed spontaneous theory of mind inferences about people with whom we are close, or whom we like, than about strangers or people whom we dislike. Situation and context are also influential motivational factors. To illustrate, skilled negotiators routinely devote significant cognitive bandwidth to figuring out what is going on in the minds of their negotiation counterparts.

While having the desire to understand the minds of others is critical to higher-level mentalizing, the *wrong* motivational impetus can have a detrimental effect on mentalization. Research has indicated that, for some people, an important motivation for strategic mentalizing is the desire to maintain rigid control over others. Such a desire can lead to *incomplete* (and hence inaccurate) mentalizing, as it directs and narrows attentional focus exclusively to social information needed for control. There are two prominent factors that lead people to employ strategic mentalizing as a means of control. The first factor is "fear." Individuals, especially those who suffer from psychological disorders such as narcissism or paranoid personality disorder, can become hypervigilant and increasingly biased in their strategic mentalizing. This fixation focuses attention toward social indicators that could indicate a *threat*. Even neutral social information could be perceived as threatening. The second factor is "reward." Some people are significantly more inclined than others to use strategic mentalizing solely for *instrumental* gain, as can be seen, for instance, in people who score high on the Dark Triad scale. Such individuals tend to lose sight of *relational* goals. The fixation on instrumental gain focuses attention toward social signals and cues that indicate an *opportunity for competitive advantage*. They ignore social indicators that would otherwise remind them to take the impact on social relationships into account.

There are two additional mental states that factor heavily into our motivation for strategic mentalizing. The first is the mental state of "knowledge." *We need to understand how strategic mentalizing works.* The second is the mental state of "belief." *We need to believe in the efficacy of strategic mentalizing, and in our own mentalization abilities.* In short, without a solid foundation of functional knowledge, and a sincere belief in the efficacy of strategic mentalizing, the motivation to apply this valuable social tool will be low.

Well-balanced and Properly Motivated Strategic Mentalizing: Advantages, Impediments and Avenues for Enhancement

ADVANTAGES

Strategic mentalizing on a well-balanced and properly motivated basis yields many benefits. On an intrapersonal level, a well-balanced and healthy motivation to strategically mentalize about ourselves *helps us to establish a more accurate understanding of our own mental states and our reasons for behaving and reacting the way we do.* This insight leads to better self-knowledge and improved ability to make well-informed decisions. A healthy and well-balanced motivation to mentalize also helps us to recognize when strategic mentalizing is called for, and gives us more control over our attentional focus and energy levels.

Interpersonally, we see that a well-balanced motivation to strategically mentalize *improves the accuracy of our theory of mind inferences about others.* Our mentalization is driven less by our own affect, and more by reflective curiosity focused on a win-win outcome.

On an extrapersonal level, we see that strategic mentalization, based on the right motivational factors, *helps us to feel at ease and well-connected in most social situations.* Additionally, it *enhances our tendency to take the situational context into account when explaining or predicting behavior,* so our inferences will not be based on bias or stereotype.

IMPEDIMENTS

Impediments to developing a healthy motivation for strategic mentalizing exist on the same three levels. Intrapersonally, it is well established that *personality and temperament have a strong influence on our motivation to mentalize.* People who have developed an insecure attachment style as a result of dysfunctional early childhood experiences often lack a healthy motivation to strategically mentalize. Additionally, certain psychological disorders, such as autism or borderline personality disorder, can severely impede the motivation to mentalize. As with the more persistent traits of personality and temperament, our state of mind at any particular time can diminish our motivation to mentalize. For instance, when we feel down and out, we tend to become more inwardly focused.

Interpersonally, our motivation depends upon the *person about whom we are mentalizing*. When we are not able to identify with someone, or when we have negative feelings toward someone, our motivation to mentalize about them can be diminished. Conversely, when we feel threatened by someone, our motivation to strategically mentalize about them may be elevated to an unhealthy level.

On an extrapersonal level, we have seen that *contextual factors can influence our motivation to mentalize*. For instance, when working under severe time pressure, we are less inclined to think about the mental states of others. Additionally, we are less motivated to mentalize about people with whom we are not familiar, which can impede our motivation to gain the perspectives of people who differ from us socioculturally.

AVENUES FOR ENHANCEMENT

Despite the myriad factors that influence our motivation to strategically mentalize (for better or for worse), there are two practices that can help to reinforce the right motivation and cultivate a healthy motivational balance. A good starting point is to *examine our own motivation to strategically mentalize about others*. We need to consider whether our motivation has the unintentional effect of narrowing our attentional orientation and focus. Also, we should examine whether our motivation to mentalize will serve our full range of strategic objectives. The next step is to *enhance our understanding of how to strategically mentalize*. Armed with this understanding we will become more confident in our mentalization abilities, and therefore more motivated to use strategic mentalizing to achieve positive outcomes.

References

Baron-Cohen, S. (1999). *The evolution of a theory of mind.* In M. C. Corballis & S. E. G. Lea (Eds.), *The descent of mind: Psychological perspectives on hominid evolution* (p. 261–277). Oxford University Press.

De Weerd, H., Diepgrond, D., & Verbrugge, R. (2018). Estimating the use of higher-order theory of mind using computational agents. *The B.E. Journal of Theoretical Economics, 18*(2). doi:10.1515/bejte-2016-0184

Fiske, S. T., Cuddy, A. J. C., Glick, P., & Xu, J. (2002). A model of (often mixed) stereotype content: Competence and warmth respectively follow from perceived status and competition. *Journal of Personality and Social Psychology, 82*(6), 878–902. doi:10.1037/0022-3514.82.6.878

Prevost, M., Brodeur, M., Onishi, K. H., Lepage, M., & Gold, I. (2015). Judging Strangers' Trustworthiness is Associated with Theory of Mind Skills. *Frontiers in Psychiatry, 6.* doi:10.3389/fpsyt.2015.00052

SECTION IV.

STRATEGIC MENTALIZING

To Reason and Evaluate

Chapter 2.

Content Extraction

Is Fiction Really Fiction?

Most of us who read fiction are familiar with the following disclaimer:

> This is a work of fiction. Names, characters, businesses, places, events and incidents are either the products of the author's imagination or used in a fictitious manner. Any resemblance

> to actual persons, living or dead, or actual events is purely coincidental.

Is this an accurate statement? Are the events and characters described in works of fiction truly fictional, or are they based on real life events and characters? When we take a look at F. Scott Fitzgerald, writer of "*The Great Gatsby*," or his contemporary, Ernest Hemingway, author of "*The Old Man and the Sea*," we see novelists who tapped into their own psychological makeup and life experiences, or those of people close to them, to develop the personalities and backgrounds of their characters. This is not surprising, as it is easier for most people to write about something that is familiar than it is to fabricate characters and events out of thin air. Some stories, such as folk tales, are passed down orally from one generation to the next, until eventually being reduced to writing. These traditional cultural narratives do not necessarily reflect aspects of the writer, but they do reveal life experiences, social values and cultural beliefs. The race and ethnicity of the characters in a book are often a strong reflection of the writer's identity and background, as well. Certain authors base their protagonist on an alter ego of themselves. Other writers reveal their deepest wishes, fears, or secrets through the characters and events in their works. Literature is a field in which narrative sharing has become an art form. In our daily lives, however, we constantly employ narrative sharing to give form to our lives, and to help others understand our perspectives. We will now take a look at the types of mental state information that we can extract from verbal accounts.

In this chapter, *Content Extraction*, we focus on the *type* of information we use to strategically mentalize. Strategic mentalizing relies, to a large extent, on the sharing of experiences through verbal accounts. Therefore, if we want to make meaningful and accurate theory of mind inferences, *we need to understand what content to extract from such verbal exchanges*. Language makes it possible for us to share verbal representations of our mental states. A "state of mind" is the psychological state of a person, or the condition or quality of a person's thoughts or feelings, at any given time. We infer mental states through verbal and nonverbal mental state indicators. These mental state conditions have predictive or explanatory value. In other words, *they have the potential to influence behavior.*

We have previously identified four primary mental states that are commonly studied in relation to mentalization and theory of mind. They range from the "mere feeling" state of affect to the more epistemic states of desire, belief and knowledge. Because these mental states have a significant influence on one another, they need to be accounted for both individually and in relation to one another. Together, these primary mental states form increasingly complex mental states such as attitudes, motivations and intentions.

We will now examine the process of inferring each of the primary mental states, starting with affect.

Affective State Attribution

The mental state of affect has already been discussed extensively in the earlier section on affective mentalizing. In this chapter, we will focus on the aspects of affect that are relevant to strategic mentalizing. At the strategic mentalizing level, we use information about affect to draw *affective theory of mind inferences*. This use of affect stands in contrast to affective mentalizing, where our underlying objective is to empathize, show compassion, or share our own affective state in order to keep our mentalization efforts online, and to maintain or reestablish healthy relationships. As explained in the previous chapter, affective theory of mind reasoning involves consideration of the possible influences that affect can have on the epistemic mental states of desire, belief and knowledge in the formation of complex mental states such as attitudes, intentions and motivations.

Strategic mentalizing relies on cognitive reasoning to *explain past behavior* and to *predict future behavior*. This cognitive reasoning is extremely important for social survival. "Social survival" is a complex endeavor because it requires a balance between the goals of affiliation and cooperation on the one hand, and the goals of social distancing and competition on the other. Affiliation and cooperation goals help us to find friends and attain social acceptance. These goals are often, themselves, means to reaching ends that cannot be achieved without the assistance of others. Social distancing and competitive goals, on the other hand, help us to maintain distance from those who pose a threat, to achieve social standing and to exert control over our own lives. Affects (particularly social emotions) play a significant role in achieving these goals. The affiliation and cooperation motive, for instance, can be observed in social emotions such as embarrassment (feeling self-conscious, often in response to violating a social rule), love (feeling close to others), happiness (sharing positive feelings), or sadness (seeking comfort from others). The social distancing and competition motive can be observed in social emotions such as social anxiety (avoiding contact with others), anger (influencing a change in behavior of another) and contempt (distancing ourselves from others). Thus, these emotions are important indicators that reveal the intentions of others to either affiliate and cooperate with us, or to maintain distance from, or compete against, us.

Through affective theory of mind reasoning, we can also *infer social roles, power and status*. Power and status tend to give people more "emotional freedom." Therefore, a good litmus test of power and status is the degree of freedom that a person has to express feelings. People with superior power or status generally have greater liberty to express their feelings to others. People with lower power or status tend to feel more constrained in such expressions. In applying affective theory of mind reasoning, we also need to take the nonsocial function of affect into consideration. Affect has a strong influence on intention formation and follow-through. For instance, a person may intend to do something, but feel too apprehensive to act on the intention.

Studies in the field of neurology confirm the involvement of affective neural regions of the brain in predicting behavior. For instance, Hooker et al. found in their 2008 study "that neural regions related to both mentalizing and emotion were involved when predicting a future emotional response." Accurate affective forecasting enables us to predict how a likely emotional response can impact a person's intention and follow-through. Affective theory of mind reasoning also helps us to infer the moral judgments of others. Such judgments reveal the attitudes of others toward people, objects, situations, etc. They also reflect a person's level of satisfaction with the status quo. In sum, *affective theory of mind reasoning provides us with the wealth of affective information that we need in order to accurately and comprehensively mentalize about others at the strategic level.*

As previously mentioned, on the strategic level of mentalization we focus primarily on verbal expressions of affect to help us infer more complex emotions, feelings and moods. Generally speaking, however, it takes more conscious processing power to infer mental states from spoken or written language than it does to detect affect through the observation of nonverbal behavior. Within the field of natural language processing, artificial intelligence systems are being developed to process, analyze and interpret large amounts of natural language data. In our everyday dealings with others, however, we need to rely on our own judgments to ascertain the underlying affects that are being expressed in a particular narration. When inferring affective mental states, we need to keep in mind that *people rarely feel only one affect at a time*. Therefore, in most verbal exchanges, we need to interpret a "cluster" of affects, including the "valence" (negative or positive feelings) and "arousal" (the energy level of the affect) of those feelings. Additionally, research consistently shows that *affect expression is profoundly context sensitive and complex*. Thus, accurate interpretation of affective mental states requires an understanding of the situation that brought about those feelings, and knowledge of the person who is experiencing those feelings. Moreover, words that indicate affective mental states are largely subject to sociocultural interpretation differences. For instance, in more traditional cultures, affects are often expressed in terms of somatoform pain symptoms, such as back pain or a stomach ache.

Research on inferring affective mental states through verbal accounts has been based predominantly on study designs measuring inferences of affects through words that explicitly express emotions. Affective expressions are, however, largely conveyed through the narration of a situation, often with the use of "figure of speech" language for rhetorical or emphatic effect. This sort of implicit and metaphorical language needs to be interpreted in an affective manner. Affective theory of mind reasoning, therefore, needs to move beyond reliance on words that explicitly indicate affect. To illustrate, we need to be able to affectively interpret snippets of sentences such as "going through a divorce" or "interview for a dream job" without the speaker specifying any affective terms. In order to make accurate affective theory of mind inferences, we need to sharpen the affect-cause detection skills that enable us to extract language that reveals the affective mental state of the narrator, and to associate the right causal factors with those inferences. Clinical psychologists tend to be well trained in the ability to infer affective states through the interpretation of narratives that are devoid of affective labels. We now continue to discuss the second primary mental state: "desire."

Desire State Attribution

Human desires, like affects, motivate us and influence our behavior. Signals and cues that manifest desires can be *cognitive* (e.g., expressing the imagination of a desired object or status), *affective* (e.g., displaying excitement) and *behavioral* (e.g., going out shopping). Elementary desires have a strong affective component, while more complex desires involve more reasoned needs and wishes, and are therefore considered epistemic or cognitive. There are four cardinal categories of desire (Ryan, 2012):

1. Survival
2. Self-determination
3. Relatedness
4. Meaningfulness

Each category adds a layer of understanding to human drive at a fundamental level. These desires can be inferred *directly* and *indirectly* through verbal and nonverbal behavior. The four cardinal desires come from the field of "motivational psychology." They are based on the four "ultimate concerns" of *death, freedom, isolation* and *meaninglessness,* as described by Irvin Yalom (see Kesebir & Pyszczynski, 2012), and on "self-determination theory" (SDT) developed by Deci and Ryan (2012). Deci and Ryan proposed three main intrinsic needs: first, the need for *competence;* second, the need for *autonomy;* and third, the need for *relatedness.* While survival and self-determination strongly relate to our mentalization efforts aimed at competitive advantage and social distancing, relatedness connects to mentalization efforts that help enhance cooperation and affiliation. The last category, meaningfulness, relates primarily to the extrapersonal level of mentalization, wherein we look beyond ourselves and our personal interactions to understand human motivation.

In the field of human motivation, desires are also referred to as motives. The concepts of desire and motive are distinguishable, however. A desire involves something that we want to attain. A motive, such as jealousy or revenge, can be seen as a force that compels us to do something to satisfy a desire. For example, when you act out of revenge you simultaneously act on the desire to settle a score. The conceptual distinction between desires and motives is not critical here, and therefore we use the terms interchangeably.

SURVIVAL

The first cardinal category, "**survival**," involves the more biological desires that we can infer through nonsocial indicator detection of interoceptive and exteroceptive sensations. As humans, while we understand that our lives will come to an end, generally we are driven by the desire to live as long as possible. Our survival motive is evident in the efforts we make to restore equilibrium. For instance, we try to manage our nutritional level, fluid level, oxygen level and temperature level, and to alleviate pain, discomfort, or fatigue. We also need to feel safe and secure. Finally, our sex and maternal drives stem from our desire to extend our existence through procreation.

According to Yalom, these motives are the most difficult to control and are, therefore, the least subject to free will. Satisfying these desires is often the genesis of habitual behavior. Once habits are formed, they compel us to perform acts in an automatic fashion. Biological motives often operate below our conscious radar. We can, however, detect the signals and cues within ourselves and others through mentalization. Primitive survival needs are primarily detected through lower level mentalization, which focuses on observable signals and cues, and on the embodied sharing of affect and behavior. With regard to intrapersonal mentalizing, we detect survival needs largely through intero- and exteroceptive awareness. The more complex and reasoned survival needs, which rely heavily on verbal accounts, are inferred through higher-level mentalization.

SELF-DETERMINATION

The second fundamental desire that we detect through social indicators is "**self-determination**." Deci and Ryan explain that, although our lives are restricted to a certain extent by environmental and social parameters, as human beings we feel the need to carve out our own place in the world. These researchers distinguish different motives that relate to the fundamental desire for self-determination. Our desire for self-determination is evident in verbal and nonverbal behavior that indicate our "**achievement motives**." In addition, human beings have a "**power motive**" - a desire to have an impact on others. As with any desire, the desire for power is stronger in some people than it is in others. Both the need for achievement and the need for power are strongly related to our motivation for material gain, known as "**acquisitive motive**." When we are not able to reach our goals, we often react with anger and frustration, which is referred to as the "**aggression motive**." The aggression motive is also triggered when we are insulted, as insulting behavior frustrates our projection of a positive image. Curiosity also fits within the category of self-determination. It pertains to our predisposition to explore and learn new things. The "**curiosity motive**" stimulates us to experience and learn new things so that we gain a better understanding of the world around us. This, in turn, satisfies our desire to gain more control over our lives. We view the satisfaction of these desires as a way to create positive self-evaluations, which enhance self-esteem, self-efficacy and a sense of control over our lives. To infer these fundamental desires, we need to look for verbal and nonverbal indicators that reveal mental states such as goal-directedness, competitiveness and openness to new experiences.

RELATEDNESS

The third cardinal category that we can infer through verbal and nonverbal social indicators is "**relatedness**." There are three motives associated with this desire, according to Deci and Ryan. The first is the "**intimacy motive**" - the desire to be part of a family, or to have close friends, and to create a private and relaxed atmosphere in which we feel loved and socially secure. As McAdams explained (1992), "[t]he intimacy motive is a recurrent preference or readiness for experiences of warm, close, and communicative interaction with other persons." He continues, "[t]he motive is conceived as a relatively stable individual-difference variable in personality readily assessed via content analysis of imaginative narrative productions." The second is the "**motive for affiliation**," also known as gregariousness. It denotes our desire to associate with other members of a group. The third and final motive is the "**social approval motive**" - our desire to adhere to social rules and regulations that support us in gaining the acceptance and cooperation of others. To infer these fundamental motives, we need to look for verbal and nonverbal indicators that reveal mental states such as the wish to approach, the desire to know more about the other(s) and the willingness to adhere to social norms and rules.

MEANINGFULNESS

The fourth and final cardinal category of desire that we infer through social indicator detection is the transcendental motive of the search for "**meaningfulness**." Throughout history, humans have pondered the meaning of life and the reason for their very existence. Meaningfulness gives us a sense of control over our destiny, it helps us to go on during difficult times, and it provides a perspective of who we are in relation to others. According to Deci and Ryan, the quest for meaningfulness includes our "**self-actualization motive**." This term, which describes the motive to realize one's full potential, was originally introduced by the organismic theorist Kurt Goldstein (see Whitehead, 2017). Carl Rogers (1961) wrote of "the curative force in psychotherapy - man's tendency to actualize himself, to become his potentialities." Self-actualization, according to Maslow (1987), represents realization of the full potential of personal growth. Maslow placed the self-actualization motive at the pinnacle of his famous psychological "hierarchy of needs." Deci and Ryan proposed that "meaningfulness" also includes our "**self-transcendent motive**," a term first described by Frankl (1985), an Austrian neurologist and psychiatrist, and a Holocaust survivor. Self-transcendent motive is defined in the *APA Dictionary of Psychology* (2022) as "the state in which an individual is able to look beyond himself or herself and adopt a larger perspective that includes concern for others." The desire for meaningfulness can be evinced through verbal and nonverbal behavior, whereby people reveal their affiliation with a belief system, the wish for self-expression, the need to make a difference, etc. We now continue to the third primary mental state: "belief."

Belief State Attribution

The concept of belief can be defined as an *acceptance* that something exists or is true, even in the *absence of proof*. Beliefs promote trust, faith and confidence in someone or something, and they shape our attitudes and opinions. Our beliefs are more cognitive, and less influenced by affective mental states, than our desires are. Beliefs do, however, have an affective component. This becomes particularly apparent when our beliefs are challenged. Conversely, beliefs play an important role in affect-regulation. For instance, belief in an afterlife can diminish a person's fear of death. In addition, beliefs impact desires, and vice versa. In satisfying our desires, we are often confronted with an approach/avoidance conflict. When we work from an "approach motivation," our goal-directed behavior is *promoted* through the belief that *our efforts will lead to a positive outcome*. When we operate from an "avoidance motivation," our goal-directed behavior is *impeded* by the belief that *our efforts will render a negative outcome*. If we really want something, however, our strong desire can challenge (and even overcome) our self-limiting beliefs. Thus, belief is an important determinant in estimating the likelihood that a person will pursue a desired goal, and the strategies that they will employ. A belief can become a knowledge state when the believer finds verifiable evidence that corroborates the correctness of a belief. Beliefs find their origins in:

- a person's own experiences or explorations;
- the acceptance of familial, cultural and societal norms; and
- the experiences and perspectives of other people.

We will examine three different categories of core beliefs:

1. Beliefs we hold about the world.
2. Beliefs we have about ourselves.
3. Expectations that are connected to goal attainment.

WORLDVIEWS

The first category, beliefs about the world (or worldviews), reflects our assumptions about how the world works. These beliefs guide our perceptions, attitudes and behaviors toward achieving goals, including higher order goals such as self-transcendence. Worldviews are also known as values. "Values" generally guide a more intuitive, common-sense and moral approach in decision-making that is based on "sociocultural" learning. Although we are generally aware of our values, they tend to be deeply rooted, and operate below the level of conscious awareness. These values tend to surface in moments of insecurity, conflict, or crisis. In such times, we either hold on to our values more tightly, or we renegotiate their importance.

Social signals and cues that reveal worldviews in narratives and statements are:

- "**Attitudinal**" - the sharing of positive or negative views toward aspects in the world, such as politics, the environment, etc.
- "**Ideological**" - the sharing of ideas and ideals that reflect a person's values or belief system.
- "**Philosophical**" - the sharing of answers to fundamental questions about the world.
- "**Religious**" - the sharing of beliefs about practices that often have supernatural, transcendental, or spiritual aspects.

SELF-BELIEFS

The second category of core beliefs involves the beliefs we hold about ourselves. "Self-beliefs" are often influenced by our personality traits as demonstrated by the theory of "core self-evaluation" (CSE). CSE represents four stable personality traits that encompass an individual's subconscious fundamental evaluations about themselves, their own abilities and their sense of control. The concept of CSE was introduced by Judge et al. (2003). According to these researchers, "core self-evaluations is a broad, latent, higher-order trait indicated by four well established traits in the personality literature." The first trait is "**self-esteem**," which reflects our overall subjective emotional evaluation of our own worth in relation to our accomplishments and capabilities, our values, our appearance, others' opinions of us, our possessions, etc. These evaluations are either negative or positive depending on the level of self-esteem, with low self-esteem correlating with negative evaluations. The second is "**generalized self-efficacy**," which involves the extent or strength of our belief in our own ability to complete tasks and reach goals. The third is our disposition for "**neuroticism**" (or emotional stability). It involves the way a person interprets and responds to ordinary situations in their daily life. The fourth and final trait is referred to as "**locus of control**." It involves a belief that we control our own lives (an internal locus of control), which makes us feel responsible for our own decisions, or a belief that our life is controlled by environmental factors (an external locus of control), which leads us to believe in chance or fate. Our core self-evaluations largely drive our motivation to follow through on our intentions. People who have *high* core self-evaluations will *think positively about themselves and have confidence in their own abilities*. They will be more likely to follow through on what they set out to do. Conversely, people with *low* core self-evaluations will *have negative appraisals of themselves and lack confidence in their ability to reach goals*. Social indicators that reveal a person's core self-evaluations are found in statements such as:

I am loved and valued, or I feel worthless.
I like to take on new challenges, or I find it hard to tackle new projects.
I like to travel without booking in advance, or I prefer a detailed itinerary.
I decide what I want to do in my life, or I find it hard to carve out some space for myself.

EXPECTANCY BELIEFS

The third category of core beliefs involve expectancy beliefs. "Expectancy beliefs" serve as one of the core explanatory constructs underlying intentions. We choose whether to invest effort in a course of action by weighing the following expectations:

1. That we have the capacity, skills and knowledge to successfully perform the behavior necessary to reach the goal. This expectation is influenced, in part, by our core self-evaluations.
2. That our efforts will result in the attainment of the desired goals. Here we gauge the expected difficulty of achieving the goal. Our locus of control and sense of self-efficacy impact these expectations.
3. That the value of the outcome will justify the effort required to achieve it.

Indicators that reveal a person's expectancy beliefs can be found in statements such as:

When I apply myself I'll reach my goals.
I don't think the effort is worthwhile.
With the work I am doing, I should earn at least as much as my colleagues.
Maybe the problem will go away on its own.

We now move on to the fourth and final primary mental state: "knowledge."

Knowledge State Attribution

The mental state of knowledge involves having an understanding of someone or something through experience or education. Whereas a statement of belief is an understanding based upon trust or faith, knowledge requires a basis in truth. It must be verifiable by facts or experience. Knowledge is the most cognitive of the four primary mental states. People often say, *"it's not what you know, but who you know."* When it comes to strategic mentalizing we say, *"it's not what you know or who you know, but what you know the other person knows."* We need this information, for instance, to gauge how well prepared the other side is in a negotiation, or to make sure that someone with whom we work actually knows what they are talking about. We also need to establish the knowledge state of others in order to appropriately tailor the content of our messages. Throughout history, different kinds of "knowing" have been identified (Bengson et al., 2011):

1. "**Knowing that**" - knowledge by description, or knowing a concept (*What does this person truly know factually?*)
2. "**Knowing how**" - understanding how something works (*To what extent does this person know the workings of something and understand how to apply their knowledge?*)

3. "**Knowledge by acquaintance**" - knowing by relation or instinct (*How deep is this person's knowledge and how well can they generalize it to other situations?*)

We base our assumptions about what other people know upon *our own knowledge*, upon *our knowledge of other people's knowledge*, and upon *what we know regarding other people's access to knowledge*. Krauss and Fussell (1991) argue,

> that assumptions about what others know (and hence what is mutually known) are necessarily tentative and probabilistic. Because they are based on a variety of sources of information that will vary in credibility and relevance, they might best be thought of as hypotheses that participants continuously modify and reformulate on the basis of additional evidence (citation omitted).

In other words, *our assumptions are based on theory of mind inferences*. If we are unfamiliar with someone, we generally assume they know what we know. This tendency stems from our "egocentric bias" to attribute our own mental states to others. We can only determine what a person truly knows by observing them, listening to their narratives, or gaining an understanding through the experiences or accounts of others. Four knowledge dimensions that we need to infer to assess the knowledge state of other people are:

1. "**Factual knowledge**," which is a type of knowledge that refers to information that is verifiable and based on facts. It involves understanding and recalling information about specific details, events, concepts, or processes. Factual knowledge is often considered the foundational knowledge that is required to learn and understand more complex concepts and ideas. Factual knowledge can be acquired through various sources, including reading, listening, observation and research. However, factual knowledge alone is not enough to demonstrate full understanding of a topic. It needs to be applied and connected with other concepts and ideas to develop a deeper understanding. Asking specific questions related

to the relevant topic can help to establish the factual knowledge that someone has.

2. "**Procedural knowledge**," which refers to knowledge about how to perform a particular task or activity. It involves understanding the steps, procedures and techniques required to complete a specific task or activity. Procedural knowledge is often referred to as "know-how." Procedural knowledge is typically acquired through hands-on experience and practice, as well as through observation and feedback from others who are knowledgeable in the task or activity. This type of knowledge is important for developing skills, as well as for problem-solving and decision-making in complex situations. Asking someone to demonstrate how to perform a specific task or procedure, or to describe the steps verbally if a demonstration is not possible, can help establish the procedural knowledge that someone has.
3. "**Conceptual knowledge**," which refers to a type of knowledge that involves understanding of abstract ideas, concepts and relationships between them. It refers to the understanding of broader principles, theories and models that provide a framework for organizing and interpreting information. Conceptual knowledge is often considered the highest level of knowledge, as it involves critical thinking, analysis and synthesis. It requires the ability to see connections between different concepts, identify patterns and generalize information to new situations. It helps individuals to better understand the world around them and make sense of new information by relating it to existing knowledge frameworks. To assess the conceptional knowledge of a person you can ask the individual to explain complex concepts using analogies or metaphors, or engage in a dialogue by asking open-ended questions that encourage critical thinking and deeper exploration of concepts.
4. "**Metacognitive knowledge**," which refers to knowledge about the following:
   - Task requirements: Understanding the goals, objectives and expectations of a task or problem.

- Cognitive strategies: Knowledge of different cognitive strategies for learning, problem-solving and decision-making, such as summarizing, elaborating, or chunking.
- Monitoring: Ability to monitor one's own progress, understanding and performance on a task.
- Evaluation: Ability to evaluate the effectiveness of different strategies and techniques for learning and problem-solving.
- Self-regulation: Ability to adapt and adjust one's own learning strategies and behaviors to optimize learning and performance.

Metacognitive knowledge is important for developing effective learning strategies, improving academic performance and enhancing problem-solving and decision-making skills. It allows individuals to make informed decisions about how to approach new tasks or problems. To assess the metacognitive knowledge of a person you can ask them to verbalize their thoughts and problem-solving processes, discuss their goals and assess whether they set realistic goals, ask them to explain their own cognitive processes, or have them describe their learning processes.

Indicators that reveal a person's knowledge state are found in statements such as:

I understand...
I have seen...
I have been...
I have a friend who...
I read ...
I watched...
I talked to...

Inferring Complex Mental States

Building upon our discussion of the primary mental states, we will now examine the "complex mental states." We begin with an exploration of the ways in which primary mental states are woven together into the more complex mental states, such as attitudes, motivations and intentions. As an illustration, we will use an example from the field of sales and marketing.

When we want to introduce a new product, we can start by changing the *knowledge state* of the customer. We do this by explaining the functions and features of the product. We also need to create an affective impression, a positive *affective state* associated with the product. It is not enough that the customers like the product, they also have to believe that it is superior to the competitive alternatives. We build customer preference by promoting quality, value, performance, etc., in order to make the customer believe that the product is simply the best option, thereby changing the customer's *belief state*. Once the customer knows the product, has a favorable feeling about it, and believes in its superiority, we need to motivate them to buy it (i.e., *desire state*). If we have done everything right, the combination of these four primary mental states leads to the complex mental state of *intention* to buy. Let us take a closer look at the complex mental state of intention.

INTENTION

An "intention" is something that a person wants and plans to do. Intentions can be seen as self-directed instructions that a person thinks will lead to a desired outcome. Intentions often ripen into behavior, and therefore reading the intentions of others enables us to accurately explain and predict their behavior with greater precision. Sheeran and Webb posit in their 2016 article, "[i]ntention offers superior prediction of behavior in correlational tests compared to other cognitions including (explicit and implicit) attitudes, norms, self-efficacy, and perceptions of risk and severity (citations omitted) as well as personality factors (citations omitted)."

As with inferring primary mental states, the attribution of intentions is not an exact science, and therefore our predictions are not always accurate.

People do not necessarily follow up on their intentions. The failure to follow up on intentions is known as the "intention-behavior gap." Factors underlying intention formation, such as opportunity recognition, feelings about required behavior and expected outcomes, etc., reside in the primary mental states. Primary mental states also influence whether the intention, once formed, is followed up with behavior. Sheeran and Webb write,

> [a]s people strive to enact their intentions, they can face various self-regulatory challenges in aligning their thoughts, feelings, and actions with their intentions (citations omitted). Self-regulatory problems may be encountered during different phases of goal pursuit and include problems (a) getting started, (b) keeping ongoing goal pursuit on track, and (c) bringing goal pursuit to a successful close ….

For example, even though we may base our intentions, in part, upon the belief that we need to conform to a certain norm, this belief state can later be overruled by other personal beliefs. Sheeran and Webb note that "[c]onsistent with self-determination theory (citations omitted) evidence suggests that intentions based on personal beliefs about the outcomes of acting (attitudes) better predict behavior than intentions based on social pressure to act (norms) (citations omitted)." Thus, we see that subsequent beliefs can supplant beliefs that were influential during the formation of the intention. Intentions built upon strong, stable and intrinsic mental states are more likely to be acted upon. In other words, *they have a higher level of intention stability*. Sheeran and Webb explain that "accumulated evidence suggests that intention stability is the best indicator of the likelihood that an intention will be realized."

Intentions can be inferred through verbal and nonverbal goal-directed behavior.

Different goals elicit different verbal and nonverbal communication patterns, for example:

- "**Instrumental goals**" (e.g., pursuing a promotion). In the book *Close Relationships: A Sourcebook,* Burleson et al. (2000) write "[w]e frequently engage in communication designed to achieve instrumental goals such as gaining compliance (getting someone to do something for us), getting information we need, or asking for support. In short, instrumental talk helps us 'get things done' in our relationships."
- "**Relational goals**" (e.g., courting a mate). Rogers and Farace (1975) studied relational communication patterns from which relational goals can be inferred, such as:
    - "**Intimacy**" - the pursuit of intimacy can be detected in the degree of depth and breadth in communication. Intimacy usually elicits behavior that indicates trust, security, vulnerability, openness and self-disclosure.
    - "**Chemistry**" - the goal of establishing and enhancing chemistry is shown through the degree of similarity between two or more people. This can be demonstrated, for instance, by signs of agreement with each other, common interests, viewpoints, and by affection or fondness. Nonverbally, it often manifests as a high level of behavioral and affective contagion, for example, exhibiting similar paralinguistic features or mimicking another's posture.
    - "**Emotional connectivity**" - the attempt to connect to others on an affective level can involve various verbal and nonverbal displays that indicate feelings of affection, excitement and happiness (when the goal is likely to be achieved), and anger, anxiety, distress and sadness (when attempts to connect with another person are unsuccessful).
    - "**Affiliation**" - the desire for affiliation is signified by informal and open communication, whereas formal and measured behaviors reflect the wish to maintain relational distance.

  - "**Relationship balance**" - the desire to achieve balance in a relationship is manifested in communication patterns that are aimed at establishing, maintaining and restoring the balance of elements such as power, care and need in a relationship.
- "**Identity goals**" (e.g., seeking recognition). These goals are reflected in communication that supports the creation of a particular identity in the minds of others. Clothing and speaking style are often used to project a certain identity. Identity goals can be cooperative (aimed at fitting in), or competitive (aimed at creating a sense of individuality). Our identity consists of different identity subsets linked to context (e.g., personal, professional, relational, communal, etc.). Certain contexts may pit one identity against another, a condition referred to by Jung and Hecht (2004) as an identity gap. Recognition of the conflicts that are posed by identity gaps can be helpful in formulating alternative explanations for past behavior and predicting future behavior.
- "**Value goals**" (e.g., believing in the value of a healthy work/life balance). Value goals can be inferred from the way people treat each other, and through their suggestions of what they view as good or bad, right or wrong, etc. This type of communication is also used for identity formation. Values are often communicated in order to change the behavior of others.
- "**Process goals**" (e.g., wanting things to be done in a certain way). These goals are reflected in the promotion of a preferred approach over other approaches. Although it is intended as a cooperative communication strategy, it can easily become very competitive, as many people connect their self-view and identity to their process goals.

Inferring Personality Factors

Strategic mentalizing focuses primarily on intentions in order to predict or explain behavior. There are several variables, however, that factor into the formation of intentions and the follow through on those intentions, and thus add predictive and explanatory value to our theory of mind reasoning. Personality factors such as a person's temperament, personality traits, competence and trustworthiness significantly influence our intention formation and goal-directed behavior. These personal aspects remain generally consistent throughout a person's life, *providing a stable predictive and explanatory baseline for behavior*.

Temperaments and personality traits are particularly informative. "Temperaments" lay the basic foundation for our personality. Our personality is shaped by the dynamic interplay between our temperament and the sociocultural context of our upbringing and experiences in life. Personality consists of different traits. These "personality traits" comprise the enduring configuration of characteristics and behavioral patterns that define our unique adjustment to life. Whereas temperament is more closely related to the mental states of affect and basic desires (drives), personality traits can be understood as particular *clusters* of mental states, consisting of affects, desires, beliefs and knowledge.

Personality traits should not be confused with personality types. "Personality types" refer to the "psychological classification" of different types of individuals. The concept of personality types is less useful for mentalization, as it lacks the specificity required to make accurate and personalized inferences. Furthermore, personality types tend to bias our perceptions of others because they lump together a predetermined set of personality traits, some of which may be present, while others are not. One aspect to keep in mind with regard to personality traits is that we tend to *overgeneralize the extent to which a personality trait is applicable to a person regardless of context*. In reality, people may use a certain personality trait in one context, but not necessarily in another. For example, we might assume that a person who is diligent in a work setting is equally conscientious at home.

As with intentions, both temperaments and personality traits manifest themselves in "natural language use." Armed with the wealth of content from social networking and online publishing sites, and sophisticated text analysis tools, researchers have made great strides in identifying "linguistic markers" of personality. Generally, research on word usage to estimate personality traits and infer intentions, distinguishes between:

- "**content words**" such as nouns (bird, Tom, flower), verbs (sing, exist, develop) and adjectives (cold, sweet, green); and,
- "**function words**," such as pronouns (I, you, he), interjections (okay, bye, huh, cool, ouch) and adverbs (quickly, beautifully, firmly).

While content words indicate *what* a person says, function words express *how* a person gets a message across, otherwise known as "language style." Ireland and Mehl (2014) argue that "individual differences in language style are often more psychologically telling and psychometrically parsimonious than are differences in language content." Therefore, function words are more indicative of a person's personality. These researchers also suggest that *function* words used in natural language directly reflect social cognition as they "require common ground or shared social knowledge to be interpreted." The analysis of pronouns, for instance, is very useful for strategic mentalizing. To illustrate, the use of first-person singular pronouns (I, me, my) suggests a focus on the self, and an increased self-awareness. The use of second-person pronouns like "you" and "you are" are often indicative of the blaming of others, a behavior particularly associated with narcissistic personality disorder. People also use pronouns as a "linguistic strategy" to promote either affiliation and cooperation or distancing and competition. The use of the first-person plural pronoun "we" is associated with affiliation and cooperation. The use of the third-person plural pronoun "they" is often used to distance oneself from others. Interestingly, when we listen to narratives of others, we generally process the pronouns used in verbal accounts *unconsciously*. Because of this, our evaluations of others, and our interactions with them, are influenced without any conscious awareness on our part of the impact of pronoun usage. Let us look at a few studies that illustrate the link between language usage and personality. We will focus in on research regarding the five broad dimensions that are commonly used to describe personality: extraversion, agreeableness, neuroticism, openness and conscientiousness.

EXTRAVERSION

"Extraversion" is characterized by "an orientation of one's interests and energies toward the outer world of people and things rather than the inner world of subjective experience" (*APA Dictionary of Psychology*, 2022). Extraversion is one of the most predictable personality traits. Mehl and Ireland (2014, p. 214; see also Yarkoni, 2010) reported that extraversion was positively correlated with the use of:

- Second-person pronouns, such as "you" and "your"
- First-person plural pronouns, such as "we" and "us"
- Positive emotion words, such as "adorable" and "nice"
- Social words, such as "party" and "crowd"
- Words referring to leisure, such as "restaurant" and "dancing"
- Words referring to sex, such as "kissed"

They also reported that extraversion was negatively correlated with the use of:

- Words that relate to inhibited behavior, such as "careful" and "avoid"
- Words that show tentativeness, such as "doubt" and "maybe"

Furthermore, extraverts were found to be more talkative. Similarly, Hirsh and Peterson found in their 2009 study on the association between personality traits and language use in the production of self-narratives, that "[e]xtraversion was associated with words related to humans, social processes, and family. These findings are consistent with the fact that extraverted individuals are active social explorers." In addition, Beukeboom et al. found in their 2012 study that "the verbal style of extraverts is characterized by a higher level of abstract interpretation, whereas introverts tend to stick to concrete facts."

AGREEABLENESS

"Agreeableness" is described by the *APA Dictionary of Psychology* (2022) as "the tendency to act in a cooperative, unselfish manner, construed as one end of a dimension of individual differences (agreeableness vs. disagreeableness)." Ireland and Mehl explain that "[a] clear and intuitive indicator of agreeableness is linguistic positivity." They reported that agreeableness was positively correlated with the use of:

- First-person singular pronouns, such as "I" and "mine"
- Words indicating positiveness, such as "wonderful" and "beautiful"
- Social words, such as "visiting" and "together"
- Words referring to home, family, friends
- Words referring to communication

They also found that agreement was negatively correlated with the use of:

- Words that relate to death, such as "coffin" and "killer"
- Words that relate to money
- Swear words/insults, such as "damn" and "jerk"

First-person singular pronouns were used by agreeable people as a "polite hedge phrase" (I think that ...) rather than reflecting "neurotic self-consciousness." The absence of the use of swear words is a clear linguistic marker for agreeable people. Hirsh and Peterson found similar results in their 2009 study. Moreover, they reported that "[h]ighly agreeable people were also less likely to use body-related words." These scholars also discovered in their research that "[i]t appears that agreeable individuals have a greater sense of certainty in their lives, and consequently think in more concrete terms."

NEUROTICISM

"Neuroticism" is, according to the *APA Dictionary of Psychology* (2022), "characterized by a chronic level of emotional instability and proneness to psychological distress." With regard to the trait of neuroticism, Ireland and Mehl (2014) indicate that people who score low on emotional stability use more:

- First-person singular pronouns, such as "I" and "me"
- "Negative emotions" words, such as "annoying" and "depressing"
- Swear words, such as "fucking"

People with low emotional stability use more negative words like "I hate" and "I am sick of," but this behavior is more generally observed in private than in public settings, as the expression of negative emotion is generally seen as socially undesirable or inappropriate. These researchers, therefore, point out that "private but not public negative emotions word usage reflects increased neuroticism." Additionally, Hirsh and Peterson (2009) found that,

> neurotic individuals were more likely to discuss body-related topics. This may indicate the increased prevalence of physical problems in neurotic individuals (citation omitted), or the fact that "body dysmorphia" (a mental health disorder whereby a person is preoccupied with an imagined physical defect or a minor defect in their appearance) is closely associated with this trait (citation omitted).

Hirsh and Peterson added that people who score high on the neuroticism scale focus in their narrative more on their home environment than on their work environment when discussing past and future events, perhaps because the work environment is perceived as a stressful place and talking about work-related experiences feels uncomfortable.

OPENNESS

"Openness," according to the *APA Dictionary of Psychology* (2022), "refers to individual differences in the tendency to be open to new aesthetic, cultural, or intellectual experiences." Ireland and Mehl (2014) explain that "openness is relatively difficult to capture linguistically." They did, however, note that "linguistic indicators of openness seem to reflect only its intellectual aspects, ignoring facets related to artistic expression and emotionality." Yarkoni (2010) found that people high in openness do not tend to use words that refer to home, family, or leisure. The research further notes that "[o]n Facebook they frequently use words like universe, writing and music (citation omitted)." According to Yarkoni, these people "adopt a more formal rather than a narrative writing style." The personality trait of openness is difficult to predict from speech, and it is more present in a person's interest in a broad array of subjects such as art, literature, travel, etc. Hirsh and Peterson found in their 2009 research that openness "was most strongly related to a greater prevalence of perceptual processes, including words related to hearing and seeing."

CONSCIENTIOUSNESS

The personality trait of "conscientiousness" is defined in the *APA Dictionary of Psychology* (2022) as the "tendency to be organized, responsible, and hardworking." According to Mehl and Ireland (2014), language of people who score high on conscientiousness, as with agreeableness, takes the form of politeness. These scholars explain that "[c]onscientiousness is best defined by the words that people high on the trait do not use." They are less likely to use swear words or references to negative emotions like "boring" or "frustrating." Phrases strongly associated with conscientiousness such as "ready for," "to work" and "great day," likely suggest the willingness to start whatever needs to be done. In addition, Hirsh and Peterson (2009) found that "[c]onscientiousness was associated positively with achievement and work-related words. Negative correlations were observed for death and body-related words."

MENTAL HEALTH AND PERSONALITY DISORDERS

Content and function words in language can also be associated with mental health and personality disorders. Not surprisingly, studies have found that people who suffer from depression make more references to negative emotions and fewer to positive emotions. Mehl and Ireland (2014) write, however, that depressed individuals may "mask negative emotions in order to maintain their social network." In addition, according to Mehl and Ireland, these people are more self-focused, and this is reflected in their higher use of first-person singular pronouns, "especially the use of I-words such as I, I'm, I'll."

We can also, to a certain extent, infer indicators of the Dark Triad from word usage. As explained in our earlier section on affective mentalizing, machiavellianism is characterized by strategic deception and manipulation of others, narcissism is characterized by self-laudatory and self-aggrandizing views, and psychopathy is characterized by disregard for others and lack of guilt or remorse.

Machiavellianism, as explained by Mehl and Ireland, positively correlates with the use of I-words and negatively correlates with the use of you, or they, words. However, when these individuals revert to impression management (attempting to control and influence the impressions others have of them) the correlation with the use of first-person singular and second-person pronouns turns around.

Mehl and Ireland tried to find a conclusive answer on the question whether "narcissism is characterized by a pervasive self-focus in social interactions and [whether] this is reflected in the increased use of I-words and decreased use of we-words." Studies have not, thus far, found corroboration for the suggestion that the use of I-words indicates narcissistic traits in people. Mehl and Ireland describe that:

> The I-use with women is more connected to anxiety and depressive symptoms than it is to any facet of narcissism. Narcissism in general, especially its "toxic" components of superiority/arrogance and exploitativeness/entitlement, was correlated with a more frequent use of swear and anger words. Narcissistic individuals make more sexual references in their daily language use.

Hancock, Woodworth and Boochever, in their 2018 study on linguistic traces of psychopathy in email, text messaging and Facebook, found:

> In online communication people higher in psychopathy, in comparison to those who are lower in psychopathy, referred less often to their conversation partner, used more psychological distancing, produced less comprehensible text, and used more interpersonally hostile language, such as anger and swear words. Psychological distancing suggests that psychopaths do not emotionally connect with what they are saying and that they are either detached from their language or use the same type of language to refer to both emotional and non-emotional concepts.

These researchers also found that people higher in psychopathy "referred significantly more to their basic needs in their [verbal] narratives, however, not in their written texts." Motivations, such as basic needs, are better elicited in verbal narratives than in written texts.

IDENTITY

In addition to using language to infer temperaments and personality traits of people, we can also use it (in combination with the information we gather through basic mentalizing) to help identify other personal characteristics. From the mere sound of a person's voice, we can infer such aspects as gender, ethnicity, emotional state, socioeconomic status, and even physical size. In other words, our identities are encoded in our speech, and our sensitivity to vocal signals can be even more accurate than our observations of someone's appearance, as Giles and Rakić (2014) explain. At times we diagnose voices, speech styles and speech content stereotypically. An accent can forge strong social judgments, and these judgments can, in turn, lead to irritation or stress and anxiety. Mehl and Ireland (2014) add that "[p]ronouns are critical in the communication of social stereotypes as they are indicative of either shared or individualistic worldviews."

Inferring Trustworthiness and Credibility

As discussed in the previous chapter, when we meet new people, we try to infer whether we can trust them by assessing their level of integrity and competence. "Deception" is an intentional act in which a sender knowingly transmits a message (verbal or nonverbal) to mislead another by fostering false impressions, beliefs, or understandings, or by actively concealing the truth. We gauge the degree to which we can trust others by their behavior and by the credibility of their narratives.

Making theory of mind inferences based on narratives requires critical thinking skills. According to Hogan et al. (2015), we need to be able to assess several aspects in the narratives of others, such as:

- The role strong statements play in an account - is it a central claim, is it a reason, is it an objection or rebuttal, or is it even relevant.
- The logical strength of inferential relationships among propositions within an argument - can you find a relationship between the central claim, the reasons or objections and/or rebuttals with regard to other aspects of the person's rationale in their narratives.
- The balance (consistency) or imbalance (inconsistency) of contrasting information presented.
- The potential for bias, for example, purposefully pitting weak arguments that lack credibility and relevance against stronger arguments.

- The possibility that information might be excluded from a narrative. Information that is intentionally or accidentally omitted can be as revealing as the information that the person shares.
- The source(s) of information presented in an argument that the person uses.

CRIMINAL INVESTIGATIONS

Let us take a look at the field of criminal investigations, where determining the veracity of statements is crucial. Making effective use of linguistic criteria for credibility analysis is an important competence in criminal justice. Determining whether somebody is lying often proves to be an extremely difficult endeavor, particularly when we have only their self-disclosures upon which to base our assessment. Both the verbal and the nonverbal indicators that have been proposed by researchers as being indicative of deception are generally *weak* and *unreliable.* Moreover, in detecting deception, *nonverbal* indicators are even *less reliable* than *verbal* indicators. The reason that it is difficult to detect deception through nonverbal behavior is related to the fact that *both truth-tellers and liars generally exhibit similar behaviors under stressful circumstances,* such as interrogation. Both the truth-teller and the liar are trying to appear as honest as possible, suppressing behavior that indicates nervousness (such as fidgeting), and employing behavior that they think is associated with honesty (such as looking the interrogator in the eye). When it comes to *verbal* behavior, on the other hand, *truth-tellers and liars use very different strategies.*

When we examine research done by prominent scholars in the field of investigative interviewing and deception, we find the following differences in strategies used by truth-tellers and liars:

- Control of information and impression management that accompany lying require a high "cognitive load," which makes lying more cognitively demanding than telling the truth. *Liars work harder* to keep their stories straight and believable, and because of this, *their narratives tend to be shorter and less spontaneous* than those of truth-tellers (Debey et al., 2012; Vrij, 2008).

- In order to control and manage the information flow, *liars often prepare answers* to possible questions others might ask, as Hartwig et al. explain in their 2007 article. Because of this, liars have an easier time answering anticipated questions than unanticipated ones. This discrepancy is not detectable in truth-tellers.
- When an interviewer requests truth-tellers to report additional information after the initial narration, *truth-tellers often add new information to their initial narratives*. Colwell et al. explain in their 2007 article: "Conversely, deceivers often give responses based upon their careful lie script and do not try to answer based upon the real event; thus, they do not benefit from such retrieval cues."
- Although truth-tellers often do not narrate their story in verifiable details immediately, Harvey et al. explain in their 2016 article that truth-tellers do add more information to their narratives when the interviewer reveals that the statements will be independently verified. When this happens, *the narratives of truth-tellers will contain more verifiable details* than the narratives provided by liars.
- *Narratives of liars are less detailed* than those of truth-tellers because "memories for genuine events should contain more external-sensorial details (e.g., color, smell, taste, etc.) and more contextual details (e.g., temporal and spatial relationships). Conversely, imagination, contamination, and fabrication ought to involve less richness and fewer external and contextual details but more details derived from internally generated memories." (Colwell, et al., 2007)
- Vrij et al. explain in their 2018 article that in order to keep their stories simple, *liars are reluctant to provide information* about "an occurrence that makes a situation more difficult than necessary." And that "as a result, *truth-tellers are more likely than liars to report more complications* (emphasis added)."
- Vrij et al. report in their 2018 article that *"[l]iars may avoid providing too many core details* [emphasis added] in an attempt to minimize the

risk of presenting incriminating information (citations omitted), but may compensate this by providing peripheral details in an attempt to provide a sufficient amount of detail."

- Hartwig et al. posit in their 2014 article that *liars,* in comparison to truth-tellers, *often change their statements,* which is known as "within-statement inconsistencies." Moreover, *they try to concoct an innocent explanation* for incriminating information they know to be possessed by the interviewer.

Relating investigative interviewing to strategic mentalizing, Granhag and Hartwig write in their 2008 article that "deception research conducted so far has very much focused on the lie-catchers' strategies, and neglected strategies applied by suspects (citation omitted)." These scholars advance the argument that

> mind-reading has an important but so far disregarded role to play in the process of detecting deception, and that the reading of a suspect's mind can be improved by utilizing psychological theory on human behaviour and reasoning.

Granhag and Hartwig recognize that investigative interviewing needs to be guided by empirical evidence. They note that "[t]he findings on deception detection suggest that police officers frequently make mistakes when attempting to mind-read." They list the following examples of mistakes made by interviewers:

- Assuming that liars are more nervous than truth-tellers.
- Being too occupied with employing their own interview strategies and tactics while neglecting the strategies their suspects use to prevent getting caught in a lie.
- Projecting their own mental states onto the mental states of the suspect - a form of mentalizing by projection, rather than employing true strategic mentalizing.

- Working from a stereotypical image they formed about the suspect (i.e., a criminal mind) and simulating mental states on the basis of assumptions with regard to this stereotypical image.
- Working from "the curse of knowledge," having a strong tendency to assume that others hold the very same knowledge they do. Granhag and Hartwig (2008) explain that "[d]ue to the curse of knowledge there is a risk that the interviewer overestimates how much the suspect knows (about what [the interviewer] knows). Consequently, the interviewer might reveal too much of what he or she knows."

In the same article, Granhag and Hartwig observe "it may be that many interviewers do not even try to mind-read the suspects at their hands, and those who try are exposed to biases that might lead them astray." They propose that "we need to consult psychological research as naive mind-reading seems to be too flawed." They continue, "a mind-reading of suspects' strategies should be used in order to predict behavior, and importantly, that these predictions should be used to plan and conduct the interview." Granhag and Hartwig conclude, "[w]hen studying other domains within investigative psychology, we learn that mind-reading is considered an important, but seldom seen, skill."

Content Extraction Acuity: Advantages, Impediments and Avenues for Enhancement

ADVANTAGES

Understanding what content to look for in narratives and self-disclosures provides several benefits. Intrapersonally, *we have the opportunity to learn a great deal about ourselves* if we pay attention to our own word choice, sentence structure, figurative language and sentence arrangement. This intrapersonal mentalizing provides us with insight about our own mental states and how these states influence our past, present and future behavior. It also provides us with a better understanding of the positive and negative reactions of others in response to our behavior.

Interpersonally, we see that through the understanding of content extraction *we can enhance our ability to process verbal and nonverbal, and social and nonsocial, signals in parallel,* improving the accuracy of our theory of mind inferences. In addition, enhanced parallel processing of verbal and nonverbal indicators helps us to quickly detect inconsistencies, contradictions and omissions (e.g., discrepancies between a person's displayed emotions and their verbal accounts, contradictions in a person's beliefs and their actions, and conflicting facts within personal narratives). It also helps us to quickly gain a comprehensive image of the person with whom we are dealing and to determine whether they are being honest with us.

Extrapersonally, *an enhanced ability to extract relevant social and nonsocial content from narratives and self-disclosures enables us to put information in context.* This significantly lowers the chance that theory of mind inferences will be influenced by bias or stereotype. In addition, it makes us better able to assess the reliability of information sources. For instance, it puts us in a better position to detect the use of propaganda, or other information of a biased or misleading nature, to promote a political objective or a self-serving point of view. In this day and age, with the abundance of information that is available on the Internet, it is becoming increasingly difficult to determine what is credible and what is "fake news." Strategic mentalizing helps us to extract the content we need in order to gain the most accurate perspective of world events.

IMPEDIMENTS

A number of factors can impede our ability to extract relevant content in verbal accounts and self-disclosures. On an intrapersonal level, *a diminished capacity to decode verbal accounts can present a significant obstacle.* This can be due to deficiencies in executive functioning, such as impaired attentional focus, or working memory deficits. *Our ability to extract relevant content from narratives is further inhibited by confirmation bias,* the preprogrammed tendency of our brain to look for confirmation of perspectives that we hold about the world around us. This tendency can lead us to ignore information that contradicts our perspectives, causing us to miss out on the full picture. Finally, *some people are predisposed to focus primarily on nonverbal indicators,* and therefore they neglect the opportunity to extract valuable content from verbal accounts.

Interpersonally, *our ability to decode a verbal account is influenced by attributes of the person with whom we are interacting.* For instance, if we lack interest in someone, or we feel stressed in their presence, our attentional focus on their verbal accounts can be disrupted. Likewise, sociocultural factors, such as language barriers, can interfere with accurate content extraction. When it comes to deception detection, *faulty assumptions about dishonesty indicators can impede us from getting to the truth.*

Extrapersonally, *contextual factors can act as impediments to accurate decoding of content from verbal accounts.* For instance, language style and usage can vary widely from one sociocultural group to another, even in cultures that share a common language. For this reason, researchers have cautioned against diagnosing personality traits and disorders by using the same language criteria regardless of cultural context.

AVENUES FOR ENHANCEMENT

Mental states are rarely expressed in explicit language but are rather "uncovered" from narratives and self-disclosures, and from any accompanying nonverbal behavior. Our brain, as Hatfield et al. (1994) explain, "is very capable of both sequential and parallel processing of verbal and nonverbal informational signals of both social and non-social aspects and does this all the time, though we mostly have the feeling that we process information exchanges only sequentially." Accurate mental state inferences are generally the result of a *co-creative, iterative endeavor* involving interactional partners, as we will explain in the next chapter. How can we improve our ability to extract relevant content from verbal accounts? First, we need to *establish a baseline* of our proficiency at extracting relevant content in verbal accounts. Depending on this baseline, we might want to:

- Improve our understanding of the type of content in narratives and self-disclosures that has predictive and explanatory value.
- Explore different methods of assessing the validity of this content.
- Enhance our ability to relate this content to primary mental states and to infer complex mental states, such as intentions and attitudes, that guide people's behavior.
- Improve our ability to simultaneously detect and integrate relevant verbal and nonverbal mental state content, and to decipher inconsistencies in verbal and nonverbal behavior and contextual incongruities.
- Improve our recognition of affiliation/cooperation and competition/social distancing motivations in narratives and self-disclosures.

References

American Psychological Association. (n.d.). Agreeableness. In *APA dictionary of psychology*. Retrieved July 17, 2022, from https://dictionary.apa.org/agreeableness

American Psychological Association. (n.d.). Conscientiousness. In *APA dictionary of psychology*. Retrieved July 17, 2022, from https://dictionary.apa.org/conscientiousness

American Psychological Association. (n.d.). Extraversion. In *APA dictionary of psychology*. Retrieved July 17, 2022, from https://dictionary.apa.org/extraversion

American Psychological Association. (n.d.). Neuroticism. In *APA dictionary of psychology*. Retrieved July 17, 2022, from https://dictionary.apa.org/neuroticism

American Psychological Association. (n.d.). Openness. In *APA dictionary of psychology*. Retrieved July 17, 2022, from https://dictionary.apa.org/openness

American Psychological Association. (n.d.). Self-transcendence. In *APA dictionary of psychology*. Retrieved July 17, 2022, from https://dictionary.apa.org/self-transcendence

Bengson, J., & Moffett, M. A. (Eds.) (2011). *Essays on Knowledge, Mind, and Action.* New York: Oxford University Press.

Beukeboom, C. J., Tanis, M., & Vermeulen, I. E. (2012). The language of extraversion. *Journal of Language and Social Psychology, 32*(2), 191–201. doi:10.1177/0261927x12460844

Burleson, B. R., Metts, S. & Kirch, M. W. (2000). *Communication in Close Relationships.* In C. Hendrick & S. S. Hendrick (Eds.), *Close Relationships: A Sourcebook* (pp. 255–56). Thousand Oaks, CA: Sage,

Colwell, K., Hiscock-Anisman, C. K., Memon, A., Taylor, L., & Prewett, J. (2007). Assessment Criteria Indicative of Deception (ACID): an integrated system of investigative interviewing and detecting deception. *Journal of Investigative Psychology and Offender Profiling, 4*(3), 167–180. doi:10.1002/jip.73

Debey, E., Verschuere, B., & Crombez, G. (2012). Lying and executive control: An experimental investigation using ego depletion and goal neglect. *Acta Psychologica, 140*(2), 133–141. doi:10.1016/j.actpsy.2012.03.004

Deci, E. L. & Ryan, R. M. (2012). *Motivation, personality, and development within embedded social contexts: An overview of self-determination theory.* In R. M. Ryan (Ed.), *The Oxford handbook of human motivation* (pp. 85-107). Oxford University Press.

Frankl, V. E. (1985). *Man's search for meaning* (Revised & updated ed.). New York, NY: Washington Square Press.

Giles, H. & Rakić, T. (2014). *Social dimensions of language variation: Social causes and consequences of language variability.* In T. M. Holtgraves (Ed.), *Oxford library of psychology. The Oxford handbook of language and social psychology* (pp. 11–26). Oxford University Press.

Granhag, P. A., & Hartwig, M. (2008). A new theoretical perspective on deception detection: On the psychology of instrumental mind-reading. *Psychology, Crime & Law*, 14(3), 189-200. doi: 10.1080/10683160701645181

Hancock, J. T., Woodworth, M., & Boochever, R. (2018). Psychopaths online: The linguistic traces of psychopathy in email, text messaging and facebook. *Media and Communication, 6*(3), 83-92. doi:10.17645/mac.v6i3.1499

Hartwig, M., Anders Granhag, P., & Strömwall, L. A. (2007). Guilty and innocent suspects' strategies during police interrogations. *Psychology, Crime & Law, 13*(2), 213–227. doi:10.1080/10683160600750264

Hartwig, M., Granhag, P. A., & Luke, T. (2014). *Strategic Use of Evidence during investigative interviews: The state of the science.* In D. C. Raskin, C. R. Honts, & J. C. Kircher (Eds.), *Credibility assessment: Scientific research and applications* (p. 1–36). Elsevier Academic Press. https://doi.org/10.1016/B978-0-12-394433-7.00001-4

Harvey, A. C., Vrij, A., Nahari, G., & Ludwig, K. (2016). Applying the verifiability approach to insurance claims settings: Exploring the effect of the information protocol. *Legal and Criminological Psychology, 22*(1), 47–59. doi:10.1111/lcrp.12092

Hatfield, E., Cacioppo, J. T., & Rapson, R. L. (1994). *Studies in emotion and social interaction. Emotional contagion.* Cambridge University Press; Editions de la Maison des Sciences de l'Homme.

Hirsh, J. B., & Peterson, J. B. (2009). Personality and language use in self-narratives. *Journal of Research in Personality, 43*(3), 524–527. doi:10.1016/j.jrp.2009.01.006

Hogan, M. J., Dwyer, C. P., Harney, O. M., Noone, C. & Conway, R. J. (2015). *Metacognitive skill development and applied systems science: A framework of metacognitive skills, self-regulatory functions and real-world applications.* In A. Peña-Ayala (Ed.), *Metacognition: fundaments, applications, and trends: A profile of the current state-of-the-art.* (pp. 75-106). Springer International Publishing Switzerland. doi:10.1007/978-3-319-11062-2

Hooker, C. I., Verosky, S. C., Germine, L.T. Knight, R.T., & D'Esposito, M. (2008): Mentalizing about emotion and its relationship to empathy. *Social Cognitive and Affective Neuroscience, 3*(3), 204–217. doi: 10.1093/scan/nsn019

Ireland, M. E., & Mehl, M. R. (2014). *Natural language use as a marker of personality.* In T. M. Holtgraves (Ed.), *Oxford library of psychology. The Oxford handbook of language and social psychology* (pp. 201–218). Oxford University Press.

Judge, T. A., Erez, A., Bono, J. E., & Thoresen, C. J. (2003). The Core Self-evaluations Scale: Development of a measure. *Personnel Psychology, 56*(2), 303–331. doi:10.1111/J.1744-6570.2003.Tb00152.X

Jung, E., & Hecht, M. L. (2004). Elaborating the communication theory of identity: Identity gaps and communication outcomes. *Communication Quarterly, 52*(3), *265-283. doi:10.1080/01463370409370197*

Kesebir, P. & Pyszczynski, T. (2012). *Motivation, personality, and development within embedded social contexts: An overview of self-determination theory.* In R. M. Ryan (Ed.), *The Oxford handbook of human motivation* (pp. 43-64). Oxford University Press.

Krauss, R. M., & Fussell, S. R. (1991). Perspective-taking in communication: Representations of others' knowledge in reference. *Social Cognition, 9*(1), 2–24. doi:10.1521/soco.1991.9.1.2

Maslow, A. H. (1987). *Motivation and personality* (3rd ed.). Harper & Row Publishers.

McAdams, D. P. (1992). *The intimacy motive.* In C. P. Smith, J. W. Atkinson, D. C. McClelland, & J. Veroff (Eds.), *Motivation and personality: Handbook of thematic content analysis* (pp. 224–228). Cambridge University Press. https://doi.org/10.1017/CBO9780511527937.016

Rogers, C. R. (1961). *On Becoming a Person: A Therapist's View of Psychotherapy* (pp. 350-1). Houghton Mifflin, Boston.

Ryan, R. M. (Ed.). (2012). *The Oxford handbook of human motivation.* Oxford University Press.

Sheeran, P., & Webb, T. L. (2016). The intention-behavior gap. *Social and Personality Psychology Compass, 10*(9), 503–518. doi:10.1111/spc3.12265

Vrij, A. (2008). *Wiley series in the psychology of crime, policing and law.Detecting lies and deceit: Pitfalls and opportunities (2nd ed.).* John Wiley & Sons Ltd.

Vrij, A., Leal, S., & Fisher, R. P. (2018). Verbal deception and the model statement as a lie detection tool. *Frontiers in Psychiatry, 9*(492). doi:10.3389/fpsyt.2018.00492

Whitehead, P. M. (2017). Goldstein's self-actualization: A biosemiotic view. *The Humanistic Psychologist,* 45(1), 71–83. https://doi.org/10.1037/hum0000047

Yarkoni, T. (2010). Personality in 100,000 Words: A large-scale analysis of personality and word use among bloggers. *Journal of Research in Personality,* 44(3), 363–373. doi:10.1016/j.jrp.2010.04.00

SECTION IV.

STRATEGIC MENTALIZING

To Reason and Evaluate

Chapter 3.

Perspective Gaining and Shifting

The Perspective of a Tribe in Papua New Guinea

The following anecdote describes the experience of a development worker in Papua New Guinea. One of the development worker's assignments was to increase the living standards of a particular tribe. In order to promote this objective, he was provided with financial means to address the needs of the tribe. When the development worker arrived, he immediately noticed that people lacked the facilities necessary for a hygienic living environment.

However, he decided to do more qualitative research to see if the tribe had even more urgent needs. The development worker designed some observation strategies to help him understand the needs of the tribal members. After concluding the observation process, he prepared an overview of the tribe's various needs. When he shared the overview with members of the tribe, they asked him to add one entirely unexpected item to their list of needs: a musical instrument for the tribal band. Although the development worker assumed that a musical instrument would not ultimately be viewed by the tribe as an urgent need, he decided to include it with the other items that would be put to a vote. His assumption proved to be very wrong, however, as a majority of votes were cast by tribal members *in favor* of a new band instrument. Concerned that he would have a difficult time justifying the expenditure to the project benefactors, the development worker tried desperately to get the tribal members to change their minds. He vigorously argued that showers and toilets, or a schoolhouse, would be of much more value to the tribe, all to no avail. The development worker was left with the unenviable task of convincing the benefactors that the project funds should go to a new instrument for the tribal band. Before he could do this, however, he needed to gain the tribe's perspective on the importance of a new instrument. After conducting more detailed interviews and listening to the narratives of the tribal members, he came to understand that the tribe's band regularly competed with the bands of other tribes. Having the best band was an important factor in keeping young tribal members within the tribe, something that was crucial to the very survival of the tribe. A new instrument would create a competitive advantage over the other tribes. Armed with this new insight, the development worker truly understood the importance of the new musical instrument *from the tribe's perspective*, and he was able to present the expenditure as an existential need.

This story illustrates the evolution from perspective *taking* to perspective *gaining*. The process starts with perspective taking through information gathering at the basic mentalizing level, and progresses to perspective gaining through the exchange and evaluation of verbal information at the strategic mentalizing level. This anecdote further illustrates the concept of perspective shifting, which involves overcoming our tendency to substitute (take) our own perspective as a proxy for the perspectives of others. Here, we step away from an egocentric perspective and toward an other-centric perspective. In this chapter - *Perspective Gaining and Shifting* - we examine how we identify and gather primary mental state indicators to form theoretical models of the complex mental states of others. We also examine the concept of perspective shifting through our ability for attributional complexity, which is pivotal to determining the most probable predictions or explanations of behavior. Let us start by examining the process of perspective gaining.

Perspective Gaining

There are two approaches to inferring the perspective of another person: One is *visual* perspective taking, and the other is *conceptual* perspective gaining. "Visual perspective taking" involves following physical changes in another person relative to their surroundings, taking their vantage point, while looking for emotional clues about the situation in their reactions (especially in their facial expressions). We use these clues not only to infer mental states, but also to regulate our own behaviors toward environmental objects, persons and situations, a process known as "social referencing." Visual perspective taking is closely related to "joint attention," which involves the shared focus of two individuals on an object or event. Joint attention is a key aspect of lower level mentalizing, during which two important skills come together:

1. following eye gaze, pointing, or other verbal or nonverbal indicators of attention, and

2. inferring mental states in the observer related to what is being observed.

The second approach, "conceptual perspective gaining," can be defined as the ability to comprehend and share the viewpoint of another person, generally as provided by the other person through verbal or written accounts. This involves higher-level mentalizing. Conceptual perspective gaining is a *gradual* and *interactive* process by which we gather information about increasingly complex mental states of another person and combine it with social information that we already know about the person (or about people in general), while taking contextual and situational factors into account.

Perspective taking and gaining are not without their challenges. One major limitation is the *tendency of humans to rely on their own perspectives in attributing perspectives to others*. Apperly (2010), for instance, states that people "often begin with their own feelings, beliefs or knowledge and adjust effortfully towards those of the target person they are supposed to be judging. This is thought to result in egocentric reasoning biases." "Perspective shifting," the capacity to rotate different perspectives in one's mind, is therefore a *critical requisite competency* for achieving accurate theory of mind inferences. We will delve further into perspective shifting later in this chapter, but for now we will focus on perspective gaining.

Gaining the perspectives of others involves the *extraction of social signals and cues that are indicative of increasingly epistemic and complex mental states*. These social signals and cues are largely revealed in the content of narratives and self-disclosures. Let us take a closer look at how these two rich repositories of mental state indicators help us to gain the perspectives of others.

Narrative Sharing and Self-Disclosure

"Narratives" are spoken or written accounts of connected events. In other words, narratives are used to tell stories. They can take many forms, such as anecdotes, fables, fairy tales, biographical accounts, etc. We do not necessarily use narratives with the intention of revealing information about ourselves, but the way we narrate our stories, and the kind of information we include, does expose a great deal about us. A significant feature of narratives is that they provide a "logical framework" for understanding motivation and behavior. Storytelling is critically important in helping us to make sense of our lives. Narratives are embedded in, and reflect, the sociocultural setting. This makes narratives crucial to the process of gaining an understanding of cultural practices, and to place the thoughts, affects and behavior of the narrator in proper context. Narratives provide insight into our interests and preferences. They guide and shape perspectives and behavior, both our own and those of others. In the previous chapter, we noted that narratives are associated with personality traits. For example:

1. Sharing complex narratives is positively associated with openness to experience.
2. Emphasizing communal involvement in narratives is positively associated with agreeableness.
3. Emphasizing negative events is positively associated with neuroticism.

The *linguistic style* and *narrative content* of the narration determine, in large part, the personality aspects that we attribute to the narrator. We employ narrative sharing on a daily basis to give form to our lives, and to help others understand our perspectives. Walter Fisher, a professor in the field of communication, built a theory on narrative sharing, which he called "narrative paradigm." Fisher's theory posits that humans are essentially "homo narrans," people who communicate primarily through narrative. As explained in his 1984 article, "[b]y 'narration,' I refer to a theory of symbolic actions (words and/or deeds) that have sequence and meaning for those who live, create, or interpret them (p. 2)." Fisher argues that it is storytelling, not rationality and argumentation, that allows the listener to participate in meaning formation. Fisher's narrative paradigm theory offers a viable instrument for content analysis. It has been applied to domains ranging from organizational communication to family interaction in therapy settings. For instance, it has been used in voter focus group research to evaluate the persuasiveness of messages in presidential campaigns. Narrative paradigm theory is also used to enhance multi-sociocultural working relationships. Encouraging employees to share stories about their sociocultural backgrounds fosters understanding, acceptance and trust among co-workers.

Narratives have features that are both intrapersonal (making sense of our own lives) and interpersonal (sharing our views with others). They are commonplace in everyday communications, but also in professional settings such as psychotherapy. For instance, research indicates that the way married couples describe their relationship in couples therapy is associated with the overall well-being of their relationship, and is, to a large extent, predictive of future divorce. A narrative therapy movement was started in the late 1980s by psychologist Dan P. McAdams in collaboration with psychotherapists Michael White and David Epston. Research on the dialogical self by Dutch psychologist, Hubert Herman, sparked further interest in narrative therapy. Narrative therapy focuses on stories people tell about past experiences that were meaningful or life changing. Significant narratives, positive or negative, ultimately shape a person's identity. McAdams and McLean (2013) describe this as a narrative identity, which "is a person's internalized and evolving life story, integrating the reconstructed past and imagined future, to provide life with some degree of unity and purpose." Narrative therapists work to change people's life stories to make those stories more understandable and acceptable, so that past negative experiences do not interfere with positive experiences in the future. McAdams and McLean further explain that "[r]esearch into the relation between life stories and adaptation shows that narrators who find redemptive meanings in suffering and adversity, and who construct life stories that feature themes of personal agency and exploration, tend to enjoy higher levels of mental health, well-being, and maturity." With regard to strategic mentalizing, of special importance is *our aptitude to infer hidden meaning or inconsistencies in narratives*. To illustrate, psychotherapists often highlight inconsistencies and conflicts in the narratives of their clients to offer insight into their conditions. Narratives that are shared during psychotherapy contain a high level of self-disclosure. "Self-disclosure" is the second core perspective sharing practice. As Duck & Usera (2014) explain, "[w]hen [we] begin to get to know each other, [we] develop a sense of relational history." Duck & Usera argue that "[a] major element of our relating with others is that we build relational history by learning about each other through self-disclosure ...." We self-disclose when we communicate with others to reveal personal or private information about ourselves. We can give a broad account about ourselves or our experiences, or we can deepen our self-disclosure by revealing more sensitive details. The information can be descriptive, explanatory or evaluative, and can include the disclosure of a wide range of mental states such as affects, beliefs, intentions, preferences and dislikes. Narratives and self-disclosures are closely linked, since self-disclosure is, in general, embedded in narratives to depict the context of what we reveal about ourselves. Accordingly, the terms are often used interchangeably.

In the early days of psychotherapy, it was assumed that a failure to self-disclose could lead to psychological problems. More recent studies show, however, that an inability to self-disclose to others is more often the *result, rather than the cause,* of psychological problems. Without question, competency in both *relating* and *eliciting* self-disclosures is critical for mentalization. Appropriate self-disclosure is often rewarded with understanding and support from others. Likewise, the more we know about others, the better able we are to understand them and offer assistance, if needed. Choosing the right time, place and audience for our self-disclosures is equally important. Self-disclosure can be very beneficial when shared with a trustworthy confidant under the appropriate circumstances. Sharing personal information with the wrong person, or in the wrong context, can be very costly. Derlaga and Berg (1987, p. 4) note that research has delineated three possible dynamics that promote self-disclosure:

1. The trust-liking approach. In general, when someone receives self-disclosure, it increases trust in, and liking for, the discloser. The recipient is then expected to return disclosure to display these feelings as a demonstration that the recipient trusts or likes the discloser.
2. The influence of social norms, similar to those of equity. Self-disclosure can be assessed by an analysis of costs and rewards, since reciprocal and appropriate self-disclosure is expected.
3. The result of "modeling," imitating the discloser due to behavioral contagion.

Self-disclosure is rule-bound, although different contexts and cultures may call for different rules. Derlaga and Berg explain that the process of self-disclosure is influenced on a moment-to-moment basis by:

- How people interact
- What an individual self-discloses
- How the recipient of the disclosure reacts
- How the discloser processes the reaction

In general, the process that promotes successful self-disclosure is comprised of the following dynamics:

- The parties create an environment that facilitates open-hearted conversations.
- Guided by basic mentalizing competencies, they synchronize their behavior with each other to establish rapport. They may begin with "small talk" to find a common ground from which they can take the conversation to the next level. One party discloses information about

himself, which invites the other to do the same. Inquiries are made in a welcoming and nonjudgmental fashion, showing the genuine desire to gain the other's perspective.

- Both parties adjust their verbal and nonverbal communication styles and messaging content to enhance connectedness and maintain conversational flow, both of which help to establish mutual trust and understanding.
- The parties may resort to unsynchronized communication, however, as a means of communicating differences and creating distance. For instance, a psychologist sometimes needs to rechannel a client's disclosure as a way of maintaining professional boundaries, so as to avoid "transference," a phenomenon in which the client redirects feelings he or she has for a significant person toward the therapist.
- The parties employ empathic and compassionate behavior in discussing sensitive topics, in accordance with sound affective mentalizing.
- Throughout the process, both parties monitor the effectiveness of their behavior, using their basic and affective mentalizing faculties.
- Both parties employ self-regulation strategies in order to stay in the present moment, keeping their mentalization faculties online, and their inferences free of bias and misunderstanding.
- The parties conform to conversational rules of propriety and accommodate each other in a colloquy of reciprocal self-disclosure.

The exchange of perspectives resulting from this process informs the parties' higher-level strategic mentalizing activities. Let us take a closer look at how narratives are decoded.

Decoding Narratives

In general, we decode narratives by paying close attention to what is being said, how it is said, and behavior accompanying the narrative. Based on the information extracted, we infer mental states, and embed them in context. Predicting and explaining behavior through narratives can be accomplished with or without making theory of mind inferences. The non-mentalistic process of inferring intentions can be likened to Silvan Tomkins (1987) "script theory." Tomkins proposed that, due to the stereotyped sequence of human behavior, action (and the expected affective states related to these actions) generally falls into patterns. Tomkins called these behavioral patterns "scripts," because they function the way a written script does, providing a program for the movement, actions and dialogue of people involved. A script is a mental construct similar to a "schema" (knowledge objects and the relationships they have with other objects, situations, or events), but which consist of a sequence of actions or events necessary to achieve a goal. Using script theory, we predict or explain behavior through a set of expectations that we have about *familiar, well-understood situations.* We create a mental picture of these action sequences, including the participants and objects involved. Script theory proposes that we create scripts for two reasons:

1. To establish or maintain cooperative and harmonious relations with others - the "**affiliation function**."
2. To compete with others for instrumental goals, social status, power, etc. - the "**social distancing function**."

We strategically mentalize about others for the same reasons. The process described by script theory is, however, clearly distinguishable from strategic mentalizing. As Schank and Abelson (1977) explain, narratives are structured in the form of scripts that consist of an ordered set of events. Because of this structure, as long as we are familiar with the scripted event, we can fill in information gaps while listening to the account. In other words, according to Schank and Abelson, the meaning of a text is more than the sum of the meanings of individual sentences. *Thus, script theory provides a useful model of understanding, at least for routine and stereotypical events.* The use of scripts is analogous to "folk" or "common-sense" psychology, which relies upon a generally shared set of beliefs to predict or explain behavior. While script theory works fine with familiar and straightforward situations, it has serious limitations when it comes to predicting or explaining more dynamic social situations. *Understanding more complex human interaction requires a mentalistic approach.* Strategic mentalizing enables us to predict or explain behavior by taking mental states into account, as well as the factors that impact these states. Strategic mentalizing closes the "information gaps" that cannot be filled in by simple common-sense reasoning or preformulated scripts. Rather than working from a script, we can tailor the inferential process to each particular situation through mental state reasoning. For instance, when a person provides an account of a straightforward negotiation, we can close certain information gaps in the narrative using our own script about how negotiations are conducted in general. If, on the other hand, it turns out that the account of the negotiation contains strange or unexpected details, we are no longer able to rely upon our "pre-programmed" script, and we need to resort to mentalization to make sense of the narrative. Predictions or explanations of behavior on the basis of script theory (or common-sense psychology) are based on how we think a person ought to behave under the given circumstances. Strategic mentalizing enables us to reach theory of mind inferences in a *systematic* and *objective* fashion. Still, scripts supply important behavioral guidelines, as without them, common social situations would be confusing and unpredictable. In complex situations, however, predictions and explanations based on scripts will generally fall short. When a situation becomes more complex, our theory of mind reasoning will produce much more accurate predictions (and explanations) than we could possibly derive from scripted "common-sense" reasoning alone.

The most rigorous method of evaluating situations is provided by the Bayesian network model. "Bayesian network models" entail probabilistic models that define relationships between variables, and can be used to calculate probabilities. Although a detailed explanation of this methodology is beyond the scope of this chapter, a general overview is nonetheless instructive.

The probabilistic technique of Bayesian network models is used extensively in the field of diagnostic medicine. Recently, it has been explored in the field of criminal justice as a method of representing and evaluating intentions. Vlek et al. proposed in their 2013 article that Bayesian networks can be constructed from "critical narrative content." This technique makes it possible to quantify how various mental states interact with the environment to form accurate theory of mind inferences about intentions. The emerging use of Bayesian networks in connection with strategic mentalizing is still being investigated. One difficulty in extending the technique to strategic mentalizing is that quantification of mental states is not as straightforward as the quantification of symptoms in the field of medical diagnostics. Bayesian network models are used in the field of medicine to determine the most probable disease given a set of symptoms. Unlike the relatively structured world of medical diagnosis, strategic mentalizing deals with a wide range of human behaviors and variable determinants. Nevertheless, the network can be used to compute probabilities of the presence of various intentions. The Bayesian network model can be employed as a tool to represent available information and a model to compare intention scenarios. The resulting Bayesian network is *not* designed to provide a conclusive decision model. It can, however, be used as an *advisory tool* to evaluate alternative scenarios or predictions. Generalizations of Bayesian networks, called "influence diagrams," can be used as a conclusive decision model. These diagrams solve both probabilistic inference problems and decision-making problems. Generalizations of Bayesian networks are often used for team decision analysis, and in the field of game theory. This probabilistic technique built on Bayesian network models can help us to keep the influence of bias to a minimum, but may not always be practical in our complex daily interactions.

In conclusion, perspective gaining enables us to gather the right amount and type of mental state information from which we can form comprehensive theories of what is going on in the minds of others. Contrasting the perspectives of others with our own perspectives, or contrasting the perspectives of different people, is equally essential to reaching a high level of accuracy in our mental state inferences. Now, let us examine our capability for perspective shifting.

Perspective Shifting

"Perspective shifting" (simultaneously holding and rotating multiple views in mind) is a form of "dialectical thinking" - analytical reasoning that pursues knowledge and truth when faced with questions and conflicts. Dialectical analysis entails the consideration of multiple rationales, and resolution of conflicts among these rationales, to develop a comprehensive point of view. In using dialectical analysis to accurately explain or predict the behavior of others, we need to be able to shift our perspective from an egocentric to an other-centric view, and consider all plausible mental state inferences. With regard to strategic mentalizing, we also focus on the construct of attributional complexity. "Attributional complexity" can be defined as a psychological construct that examines the degree to which an individual seeks to understand the causes of other people's behavior, and is willing to consider many alternative explanations (see Fletcher et al., 1986). Attributions entail judgments about causes and reasons, motives and goals of action, responsibility and origins of emotions, etc. When we mentalize strategically about others, we are constantly *generating* and *updating* our mental models with the social signals and cues that we gather. We can relate this process to the "theory of predictive coding" in which available sensory input is processed by different brain regions, and which together with various neurological processes, such as working memory and critical thinking, is used to generate a mental model of what is going on. This predictive model is based in part on knowledge that one already has. It can also be viewed as a "parallel processing model" which is described by McClelland and Rumelhart (1981) as the meeting of "top-down" (conceptual) and "bottom-up" (sensory) elements. When the predictive model does not match the situation, the prediction error is registered in the neurological network, and the model is updated and revised. This is actually a form of Bayesian inference used to dynamically update the probability for a prediction as more evidence or information becomes available. Individuals who score *high* on attributional complexity scales *tend to achieve greater theory of mind accuracy, and therefore, are relatively less prone to making prediction errors.* People with a high level of attributional complexity, such as skilled social psychologists, are more likely to consider influential factors such as a person's disposition, situational aspects and past experiences. In contrast, people with a lower level of attributional complexity are found to be less likely to consider multiple explanations for behavior. Error, bias and stereotyping in forming social judgments appear to be significantly reduced in people with a high level of attributional complexity. Let us take a closer look at certain biases that can impede strategic mentalizing.

Attributional Biases

Our own perspectives and intentions impact how we encode and decode information. Consequently, the same verbal or nonverbal message may mean different things to different people. "Bias" is often at the heart of miscommunication or misperception. Common "attributional biases" that can impact mentalization include:

- The "**illusion of asymmetric insight**" - a cognitive bias whereby we tend to think that we have more knowledge about others than others have about us. "This illusion of asymmetric insight has been traced to people's tendency to view their own spontaneous or off-the-cuff responses to others' questions as relatively unrevealing even though they view other's similar responses as meaningful" (Pronin et al., 2001/2008).

- The "**correspondence bias**," also known as the "fundamental attribution error," - the tendency to default to dispositional and personality-based explanations for behavior, while ignoring situational explanations.
- The "**actor-observer bias**" - an attributional bias that is related to the correspondence bias. Here we attribute other people's behavior to internal causes (personality-based explanations), while attributing our own actions to external causes (situational explanations). Actor-observer bias refers to attributions for the behaviors of others, as well as for our own behaviors.
- The "**self-serving bias**," which is related to the actor-observer bias - the tendency to attribute positive outcomes to ourselves and negative outcomes to external factors.
- The "**egocentric bias**" - the tendency to over-rely on our own perspectives or to have an unjustifiably high opinion of our own influence and importance. The egocentric bias is clearly observable in young children before their theory of mind abilities are well-developed.
- The "**hindsight bias**," also known as the "knew-it-all-along effect" or "creeping determinism," - the tendency to think, with the benefit of hindsight, that we knew what was going to happen from the very beginning. Hindsight bias often causes us to have distorted memories of what we knew and/or believed all along. It is a significant source of overconfidence in our ability to predict the future, and can be viewed as a form of pseudomentalization.

We will now continue with an examination of two key cognitive processes that provide essential support to the perspective gaining and shifting process: "cognitive control" and "cognitive flexibility."

Cognitive Control and Cognitive Flexibility

Scientific research has indicated that mentalization abilities are strongly associated with both "executive functioning" and "self-regulation." In other words, people who score well on executive functioning and self-regulation assessments also tend to achieve high scores on mentalization scales. Let us take a closer look at both of these supportive cognitive capacities. We have divided the components of executive functions and self-regulatory functions into two categories: 1) those that are essential for cognitive control and 2) those that are essential for cognitive flexibility. Cognitive control and cognitive flexibility are equally important to well-balanced mentalizing. For example, in order to apply the right attentional focus and perspective gaining abilities we need cognitive control. At the same time, however, in order to alternate attentional focus and shift perspectives we need cognitive flexibility.

COGNITIVE CONTROL

"Cognitive control" refers to the mind's ability to create an "information picture" that guides behavior. Cognitive control allows us to stop and think, select behaviors that we find appropriate, and reject behaviors that we deem inappropriate. It also helps us to clarify our long-term goals and purposes. Cognitive control, in conjunction with our capacity for mentalization, is at the center of our sense of self- and other-awareness. It pertains to our highest level of consciousness, to our will power, and to our free will. Scientific studies explain that cognitive control is critical to bringing and keeping mentalization faculties online. Cognitive control involves executive functioning processes such as: attentional control, working memory control and self-regulation all of which are fundamental to self-regulatory functioning such as, strategic planning, goal-directedness, higher-order thinking control (e.g., systematic processing of information, comprehension monitoring) and metacognitive thinking control (e.g., taking time to think about how we think and understanding what knowledge is in general, and how we come to know things).

The "attentional aspect" of cognitive control refers to our ability to sustain attention. There are two important attentional modes: "focused attention" and "open monitoring." While focused attention helps us to concentrate on the gathering of the *core information* critical for theory of mind inferences, open monitoring facilitates the gathering of *peripheral social and nonsocial information* that adds predictive or explanatory value to theory of mind inferences.

The "working memory aspect" of cognitive control is the temporary active retention of information for concurrent, prospective and retrospective theory of mind reasoning (in other words, for mental time travel). It is a kind of "sustained attention" focused on an internal representation that will be useful in the near term. Working memory should not be confused with short term memory (i.e., memorizing a piece of information temporarily, for instance remembering a phone number long enough to dial it). Working memory is more than mere information retention. It is a system for integrating new information with stored memory to carry out complex cognitive tasks such as learning, reasoning, decision-making and comprehension. When it comes to mentalization, working memory is required to gather and keep social information online so that we can integrate mental state information into comprehensive theories of mind.

The "self-regulation aspect" of cognitive control relates to a subset of self-regulatory control processes that aim to override undesired, prepotent impulses or urges. It also encompasses affect-regulation. These self-regulatory abilities are fundamental to mentalization, as they enable us to resist distractions, keep strong emotions in check, and to respond to others in an objective and unbiased fashion. We will now continue with an examination of cognitive flexibility.

COGNITIVE FLEXIBILITY

"Cognitive flexibility" refers to our ability to disengage from a previous task, and respond effectively to a different task, or to multitask. Cognitive flexibility allows us to:

- detect changes in circumstances and redirect attention to elements that are in flux,
- recognize that a previous strategy is not appropriate in the light of new circumstances, and
- re-formulate strategies accordingly.

Cognitive flexibility is essential to keeping and rotating multiple perspectives and concepts in our minds simultaneously. It pertains to our capacity to adjust our own perspectives, and to override habitual thought patterns and behavior. Cognitive flexibility is vital to mentalizing in rapidly changing environments. As with cognitive control, cognitive flexibility is dependent on executive functioning processes involving attention, working memory and self-regulation. It is also critical for higher-order thinking flexibility (e.g., attributional complexity, conditional knowledge, debugging strategies) and metacognitive thinking flexibility (e.g., meta-strategic knowledge about different ways we can think about something, including the ability to change our thinking strategies to improve our cognitive learning style).

The "attentional aspect" of cognitive flexibility relates to our ability to alternate our attentional focus. In relation to mentalization, cognitive flexibility enables us to adjust our attentional focus to the appropriate mentalization level (basic, affective, or strategic), and to switch easily between attention modes (focused attention or open monitoring attention).

The "working memory aspect" of cognitive flexibility is essential for manipulating and reconstituting contents that we temporarily retain in our minds. Mentalization requires the capacity to rotate different perspectives in our minds, and to be able to shift from one mindset to another, which we refer to as perspective shifting.

The "self-regulation aspects" of cognitive flexibility are critical to adjusting our behavior and responses to changing situational demands. In relation to mentalization, flexibility in self-regulation refers to the breadth of regulation strategies and skills that enable us to change from one regulation strategy to another.

Perspective Gaining and Shifting Skills: Advantages, Impediments and Avenues for Enhancement

ADVANTAGES

Well-developed perspective gaining and shifting competencies yield many benefits intrapersonally, interpersonally and extrapersonally. On an intrapersonal level, well-developed perspective gaining and shifting skills in general lead to *greater self-confidence and an increased sense of self-determination in social situations*. They also help us to *see beyond our self-centric view of situations and social interactions.*

On an interpersonal level, competency in perspective gaining and shifting enables us to *use narratives and self-disclosures more deliberately to gain an understanding of the perspectives of others, and to clarify our own perspectives.* It minimizes the risk of reaching faulty theory of mind inferences due to bias. It also influences the way we are viewed by others. Research indicates that people who have well-developed perspective gaining and shifting skills are viewed as good listeners, and as being wise and mature, socially competent, empathetic and compassionate. These are the qualities of people to whom others turn for advice. People who display a high level of attributional complexity are characterized as intelligent and intellectually oriented, even though this ability is not necessarily associated with traditional measures of academic ability and achievement.

On an extrapersonal level, well-developed perspective gaining and shifting skills help us to *better understand how narratives and self-disclosures can be used to study, understand and influence larger groups of people.* They also increase our awareness of sociocultural and contextual influences on narrative sharing and self-disclosure.

IMPEDIMENTS

There are a number of impediments to perspective gaining and shifting. On an intrapersonal level we see that *underdeveloped basic and affective mentalizing competencies, along with deficiencies in executive functioning and self-regulatory functioning,* can impede processes that promote successful narrative sharing and self-disclosure. Complex social interactions, such as narrative encoding and decoding, can be cognitively demanding. It takes effort and practice to stay focused on content extraction and evaluation. Fatigue, distraction and impatience can all lead us to default to folk psychology. Preexisting biases can also prevent us from gaining accurate perspectives.

On an interpersonal level, *we cannot always rely on other people to clearly share or volunteer their perspectives.* Lack of trust or rapport can diminish the willingness of people to exchange perspectives freely. *Overlooking inconsistencies, contradictions and potential bias in the narratives of others* can also hamper well-informed perspective gaining.

On an extrapersonal level, *contextual and cultural factors may curtail perspective gaining.* Sociocultural behavioral norms and standards, in particular, can limit the opportunity to reveal personal or private information. Additionally, contextual circumstances can make self-disclosures and narrative sharing impractical or inappropriate. Needless to say, it is nearly impossible to share narratives and self-disclosures without the help of a translator when parties do not share the same language.

AVENUES FOR ENHANCEMENT

As we have discussed, the main objective of perspective gaining and shifting is to identify and gather primary mental state indicators that reveal another person's complex mental states such as attitudes, intentions and motivations. These indicators are extracted from verbal representations (and the accompanying nonverbal expressions) that often take the form of narratives and self-disclosures. Therefore, perspective gaining and shifting competencies can be enhanced through:

- Well-developed basic mentalizing skills: first, to integrate verbal social indicators with nonverbal mental state signals and cues; and second, to connect with others in a way that invites perspective sharing through narratives or self-disclosures.

- Well-developed affective mentalizing skills: first, to assure empathic and compassionate responses, and affective communication that keep the mentalizing faculties of all parties online; and second, to maintain conversational flow, especially in the face of stress, and during the sharing of relevant emotional information.
- A good understanding of the difference between perspective taking, gaining and shifting, and the ability to apply these different components of strategic mentalizing appropriately.
- A good understanding of the cognitive reasoning skills and methodologies that are critical for theory of mind reasoning, such as attributional complexity, analytical thinking and metacognitive thinking.
- Adaptable communication skills, to promote narrative sharing and iterative development of perspective insight.
- A high level of cognitive control and flexibility, to facilitate verbal content detection and parallel processing of verbal and nonverbal social and nonsocial information, to counteract the tendency to impute our own perspectives to others, to prevent bias, and to improve our capacity for attributional complexity.

ETHICAL CONSIDERATIONS

Perspective gaining and shifting often involves a *reciprocal exchange of personal and private information*, and therefore is dependent upon a *relationship of mutual trust and confidence*. With this in mind, we conclude this chapter by revisiting two relevant principles from our code of conduct:

Principle 2, which stresses that:

> In our dealings with others, we should avoid unjust practices by taking into consideration our biases, our level of mentalization competence and the inherent limits of mentalization.

Principle 4, which advocates that:

> At all times we need to respect the rights and dignity of other people, including their rights to privacy and confidentiality.

References

Apperly, I. (2010). *Mindreaders: the cognitive basis of" theory of mind"*. Psychology Press / Taylor & Francis Group.

Derlaga, V. J., & Berg, J. H. (1987) *Self-Disclosure: Theory, Research, and Therapy*. Springer Science & Business Media.

Duck S., & Usera D. A. (2014). *Language and interpersonal relationships*. In T. M. Holtgraves (Ed.), *Oxford library of psychology. The Oxford handbook of language and social psychology* (p. 188–200). Oxford University Press.

Fisher, W. R. (1984). Narration as a human communication paradigm: The case for public moral argument. *Communication Monographs, 51,* 1-21. https://doi.org/10.1080/03637758409390180

Fletcher, G. J. O., Danilovics, P., Fernandez, G., Peterson, D., & Reeder, G. D. (1986). Attributional complexity: An individual differences measure. *Journal of Personality and Social Psychology, 51(4), 875–884.* doi:10.1037/0022-3514.51.4.875

McAdams, D. P., & McLean, K. C. (2013). Narrative identity. *Current Directions in Psychological Science, 22*(3), 233–238. doi:10.1177/0963721413475622

McClelland, J. L., & Rumelhart, D. E. (1981). An interactive activation model of context effects in letter perception: I. An account of basic findings. *Psychological Review, 88*(5), 375–407. doi:10.1037/0033-295x.88.5.375

Pronin, E., Kruger, J., Savtisky, K., & Ross, L. (2001). You don't know me, but I know you: The illusion of asymmetric insight. *Journal of Personality and Social Psychology, 81*(4), 639–656. doi:10.1037/0022-3514.81.4.639

Pronin, E., Fleming, J. J., & Steffel, M. (2008). Value revelations: Disclosure is in the eye of the beholder. *Journal of Personality and Social Psychology, 95*(4), 795–809. doi:10.1037/a0012710

Schank, R. C., & Abelson, R. P. (1977). Scripts, Plans, Goals and Understanding. Hillsdale, MICH: Laurence Erlbaum.

Tomkins, S. "Script Theory". *The Emergence of Personality*. Eds. Joel Arnoff, A. I. Rabin, and Robert A. Zucker. New York: Springer Publishing Company, 1987. 147–216.

Vlek, C., Prakken, H., Renooij, S., & Verheij, B. (2013). *Modeling crime scenarios in a Bayesian network. Proceedings of the Fourteenth International Conference on Artificial Intelligence and Law - ICAIL '13.* doi:10.1145/2514601.2514618

SECTION IV.

STRATEGIC MENTALIZING

To Reason and Evaluate

Chapter 4.

Perspective Shaping

The Father of Spin

One of the most influential Americans of the 20th century was Edward Louise Bernays, son of Anna Freud Bernays, the sister of Sigmund Freud. Known as the "father of public relations," or the "father of spin," Bernays drew on the social sciences to influence and shape the behavior of public or targeted audiences, creating and defining his own "pioneering" brand of public relations in the process. To Bernays, the public was nothing more than an irrational herd, susceptible to manipulation and influence for the benefit of his clients. He promoted the use of crowd psychology and psychoanalysis to control the masses in a manner that served the objectives of influential people and organizations. He keenly understood the power of behavioral contagion, and how this tendency could be used to influence and shape the behavior of people by manipulating their mental state of desire on a subconscious level.

Bernays was heavily influenced by Freud's notion that people's behavior is ineluctably driven by irrational subconscious forces. Bernays sought to harness this power to manipulate the masses, whom he viewed as irrational, and in need of direction. He earned fame and fortune by helping organizations such as Proctor and Gamble, General Electric, the US government and politicians to influence the behavior of people for their own benefit.

In the 1920s, America was becoming more democratic and wealthier, with the result that more and more people could influence the direction of the country. Members of the "establishment" found it increasingly difficult to maintain their grip on the masses, and sought new ways to get people to do their bidding. They found in Bernays the perfect collaborator, as he understood that in order to influence the masses, you have to control their minds.

The first major behavioral influence engineered by Bernays, one that made him a leading figure in the field of public relations, was his campaign to convince women to start smoking. In the 1920s, it was not socially acceptable for women to smoke, and this social stigma prohibited cigarette companies from capturing approximately one half of the potential market. Bernays was approached by the American Tobacco Company to change this convention. In formulating his public relations campaign, Bernays wanted to understand the symbolic significance of cigarettes to women. He enlisted the services of noted psychoanalyst Dr. A.A. Brill who advised Bernays that cigarettes were symbolic of the freedom enjoyed by men. Recognizing the desire of women to gain more freedom and independence in society, Bernays devised a campaign to associate cigarette smoking with freedom. He enlisted prominent American debutants to light up cigarette after cigarette as they participated in the annual New York City Easter Sunday parade on Fifth Avenue, as an expression of their emancipation. In their coverage of the Easter Day festivities, numerous US newspapers, including The New York Times in a front-page story, reported on the young women and their "torches of freedom." Cigarette sales immediately soared.

This anecdote illustrates the awesome persuasive power of strategic mentalizing. But just as strategic mentalizing can be used to influence others, it can also be used to resist the harmful influence of others. In this age of mass marketing, artificial intelligence, disinformation campaigns and social media, the importance of understanding and employing strategic mentalizing cannot be overstated.

In previous chapters we explained what strategic mentalizing entails, and we examined its constituent competencies. In this chapter, *Perspective Shaping,* we will focus on applying strategic mentalizing efforts to increase our influential power by shaping the perspectives of others. In addition, we examine how mentalization strengthens our ability to resist unwanted influence.

The Role of Influence

As human beings, we all have a desire for "self-determination." In order to reach and maintain a healthy level of control over our lives, we need to achieve the right balance between influence tactics that facilitate affiliation and cooperation, and those that promote social distance and competitive advantage. From an evolutionary standpoint, we are all wired to manage the balance between "convergence" and "divergence" in our relationships. We converge with others for security reasons, to share in the products and services generated through cooperative efforts, and to learn from one another. We diverge from others when competing for resources, when others pose a danger to our well-being, or when others do not possess or share the experience we need. Our convergence and divergence goals dictate, to a large extent, the strategic vectors that we choose to influence others.

Well-developed strategic mentalizing enables us to *select and implement the most effective influence tactics.* These tactics are designed to adapt our own mental states, and to change the mental states of others; in other words, we use them to *shape perspectives.* "Perspective shaping" is our conscious and controlled use of mentalization to impact the mental states and behavior of other people in order to meet our objectives. This can be as simple as cheering up a co-worker, who just had a bad review, in order to refocus the colleague on the task at hand. There are four fundamental determinants that influence the dynamics of perspective shaping:

1. The person who is attempting to bring about changes in the mental states of others.
2. The methods used to bring about the changes.
3. The target (or targets) of the attempts.
4. The methods used to resist change.

We will now take a closer look at each determinant, starting with the person who is attempting to bring about changes in the mental states of others.

The Influencer

In the course of their social interactions, people reciprocally mentalize about one another, taking turns in influencing and being influenced. As long as a "healthy power balance" is maintained, the give-and-take nature of perspective shaping will yield a satisfactory result. If not, however, one party may feel overpowered by the other's influence. Finding a healthy power balance can prove to be challenging. This is due, in part, to disparities among people in the personal characteristics that are associated with influential power, such as high status, likeability and physical attractiveness. We are inclined to focus our attention on, and therefore be more susceptible to influence by, people who possess these personal characteristics. Moreover, we tend to automatically attribute a high level of competence and integrity to such people. When we perceive others as having high levels of trustworthiness and competence, we more readily yield to their influence. These positive attributions, often unsubstantiated, endow such people with greater opportunity and freedom to influence others. People who lack these positive characteristics are more likely to be ignored or discounted, and their attempts at influence are perceived by others as illegitimate. People who have a chronic sense of insignificance or inferiority typically feel that they lack control over situations. They feel as though they constantly need to fight for their rights, their space, and their interests, which can generate chronic feelings of anger, sadness and frustration. This, in turn, can lead them to employ unhealthy influence tactics such as manipulation, coercion, or deception. Resort to antisocial influence tactics is often accompanied by poor mentalization competencies, which impede the ability to form an accurate theory of mind. We also know that the experience of strong feelings and emotions can bias the way we view others and their intentions, and impact how we perceive their behavior. People who derive their influential power from positive stereotypical characteristics (physical appearance, likeability, high status, etc.) may, in fact, be less inclined to use strategic mentalizing to influence others. Such people do not need to work very hard to convince other people to do their bidding. People who do not enjoy the benefit of positive stereotypical characteristics tend to be more effective mentalizers, as they need to rely more heavily on "mindreading" as an instrument of influence. Thus, the level of "apparent" influential power that we have can impact our mentalization abilities. It can also increase or decrease our motivation to mentalize, and it can bias our theory of mind inferences significantly. Biased perspectives related to the stereotypical characteristics of others can be hard to "re-shape" without the benefit of mentalization. Let us examine the impact of bias in the context of gender inequalities.

A DOUBLE BIND FOR WOMEN

In many cultures, people continue to attribute a higher status (and a higher level of competence) to men in comparison to women. This stereotypical view leads to a significant gender disparity in perceived influential power. When a man and a woman display an equivalent level of competence, people will nonetheless tend to rate the man as being more competent, in the absence of clear and convincing evidence to contradict the gender bias effect. Carli (2017) explains this difference in influential power by the stereotypical views we have of men and women in relation to "agentic" and "communal" behavior. Men, for instance, are viewed as having more "agency," the capacity to act independently and to make their own free choices. Moreover, agentic behavior is more acceptable coming from men than it is coming from women. Women, on the other hand, are viewed as more likeable and communal (e.g., agreeable and cooperative). Being likeable and displaying communal qualities is accepted in both men and women. Men, however, are rewarded to a greater extent for communal behavior than women, as this behavior is often taken for granted in women due to gender stereotypes. Carli notes that these "[g]ender stereotypes create a double bind for women." She reasons that "[w]omen need to show a higher level of competence to compete with men, though they will be less liked and seen as more domineering and threatening." In addition, Carli notes "[w]omen need to show a higher level of communion than men to be rewarded for it, though they will be disrespected and denigrated for being weak and incompetent." In other words, when women try to *increase their influential power by raising their level of competence*, they wind up *losing* influential power because it makes other people view them as less likable. When women try to *increase their influential power through increasing their likeability and communal behavior*, their influential power *decreases* because they are seen as weaker and more vulnerable, and hence, less competent. Carli proposes "[w]omen's somewhat greater reliance on transformational leadership, which blends agentic and communal qualities, may be one way that women can overcome their perceived disadvantage as leaders and influence agents."

Changing personal characteristics in an effort to increase influential power can be difficult, or even impossible in the case of gender or cultural background. Influential power does not hinge exclusively on personal characteristics, however. It also depends on our ability to read people accurately, and to choose the right opportunities, instruments and tactics to shape the mental states of others. We will now examine the forms those influence tactics can take.

Tactics Used to Shape Perspectives

The tactics we use to change the mental states of others vary with such factors: as our goals, our preferred tactics, and the target of our influence. Influence tactics can be verbal or nonverbal. In general, the most effective influence tactics involve a combination of both. Verbal tactics, such as framing a message in a way that grabs someone's attention, can be very persuasive, but such a tactic, if too overwhelming, can also divert attention away from the central message. Nonverbal tactics, such as cadence and tone of voice, body posture and facial expressions, can greatly enhance or diminish the persuasiveness of our message.

In the *Oxford Handbook of Social Influence* (Harkins et al., 2017) the following four principal types of influence are described: conformity, compliance, obedience and self-presentation.

CONFORMITY

The first type of social influence, "**conformity**," refers to social influence involving inducement of a change in belief or behavior in order to fit in with a group. Common tactics to promote conformity include:

- "**Social comparison**," a tactic that appeals to our motive for self-evaluation and our motive for self-enhancement. This tactic is based on "social comparison theory," described in the *APA Dictionary of Psychology* (2022) as: "the proposition that people evaluate their abilities and attitudes in relation to those of others in a process that plays a significant role in self-image and subjective well-being." Comparing ourselves to others in society whom we rank higher on positive qualities such as status and power often brings about feelings of tension. This tension can translate into a desire to be more like them, with the consequence that we start to act like them. Mimicry, affective contagion and behavioral contagion can be viewed as variants of conformity that we engage in on a subconscious level. Comparing ourselves to people whom we rank lower in status can translate into a desire to distance ourselves from them through differentiating behavior and appearance.
- "**Opinion comparison**," a tactic that appeals to the motivation to understand how the world works. When we hear the opinion of someone similar to us, but who appears to have more expertise in the relevant subject matter, we more readily accept the opinion of the "subject matter expert." When the subject matter expert is very different from us, we do not tend to accept the opinion of the "subject matter expert" so easily.
- "**Ostracism**," or the threat of being ostracized, is one of the most powerful tactics of social influence. Hales et al. (2017) note that "[r]ejection is an important force behind processes such as conformity ... . Being the target of ostracism activates brain regions associated with pain, threatens fundamental needs, worsens mood, and causes behavior changes aimed at fortifying threatened needs." We use ostracism: to protect the community from members who threaten our well-being; to correct the behavior of community members who threaten group cohesion; and to remove people permanently from the group when they do not conform to the group norms.

COMPLIANCE

The second type of social influence, "**compliance**, " refers to social influence involving inducement of action in response to a request or suggestion. Buss et al. (1987) listed six compliance tactics that are used in close relationships: *charm, silent treatment, coercion, reason, regression* (reverting to immature behavior: pouting, sulking) and *self-abasement* (acting submissively to invite assistance). Later, Buss (1992) added six additional tactics found in a broader context: *responsibility invocation, reciprocity, monetary reward, pleasure induction, social comparison* (everyone else is doing it) and *hardball* (doing anything that is necessary to have others comply). Cialdini (2009), one of the world's most prominent experts on social influence, organized compliance tactics by the six classic principles of social influence: *scarcity* (limit the time that a service or a product is available, or making a service or product exclusive), *reciprocity, commitment* and *consistency* (lowball, bait and switch, and foot-in-the-door techniques), *authority* (related to obedience*), social validation* or *social proof* (related to conformity) and *liking* and *similarity*. He later added a seventh principle, *unity*. The "unity principle" is "the shared identity that the influencer shares with the influencee," which can be used as an influence tactic by appealing to another's sense of belonging (Cialdini, 2016).

OBEDIENCE

The third type of social influence, "**obedience**," refers to social influence involving inducement of action in response to a direct order, usually from an authority figure. Obedience was researched in the 1960s by Yale University psychologist Stanley Milgram. In a series of social psychology experiments, Milgram (1963) studied the willingness of participants to obey an authority figure who ordered them to carry out acts - in the form of the administration of electric shocks to a confederate "learner" - that conflicted with the personal conscience of the participants. Milgram demonstrated that most participants would give a helpless victim what they believed to be a fatal electric shock when ordered to do so by a person in a position of authority. Milgram's experiments highlighted the dangers of "blind obedience," also referred to as "destructive obedience." Obedience is a social influence that is based on the perception that a reward or punishment is, or could be, consequential to respectively obeying or resisting the influence of an authority figure.

SELF-PRESENTATION

The fourth type of social influence, "**self-presentation**," refers to social influence involving an individual's attempt, through expression and behavior, to shape how they are viewed by others. Objectives of self-presentation are fitting in or standing out, and acquisition or protection. "Self-presentation," as described in the *APA Dictionary of Psychology* (2022), is part of a broader set of behaviors called "impression management." Some common strategies of self-presentation, as defined in the same dictionary, include:

- "**Exemplification**" - a strategy for self-presentation that involves a person's attempts to project an image toward others of a virtuous person whose behavior is consistent with the positive shared values of the group, community or culture.
- "**Self-promotion**" - a strategy of making oneself look good to others by highlighting or exaggerating one's competence and abilities.
- "**Supplication**" - a strategy for self-presentation that involves depicting oneself as weak, needy, or dependent so as to motivate others to provide assistance or care.

INFLUENCING MENTAL STATES

Influence tactics need to activate the proper affect (feeling, mood, or emotion) to motivate the intended changes. For instance, anger will trigger a different behavioral response than sadness or worry. There are different affective clusters that we can tap into in our attempts to influence others:

- "**Trust**," a feeling of safety that underlies the reliance on, or confidence in, the dependability of someone or something, heavily influences our behavior. Trust is often leveraged as an instrument of influence by people who understand that we are reliant on them for their expertise and competence. They know that trust diminishes our vigilance, which can often lead to blind reliance.

- "**Happiness**" and "**contentment**" are used to induce the belief that these positive feelings will result if we do what the influencer advises us to do. While eliciting happiness is best approached through active influence tactics (offering a reward), contentment is best elicited through passive influence tactics (promising stability and security).
- Negative feelings of "**fear**," "**anxiety**" and "**worry**" are powerful affects that can be leveraged as instruments of influence. These feelings make us want to protect ourselves (including our possessions), or to protect others. Arousing fear, anxiety and worry is an effective tactic if the target of influence is actually capable of doing something to mitigate the risk. The anticipation of a lowered level of anxiety can be used as an influence tactic by appealing to positive feelings of security.
- Three moral emotions - "**anger**," "**contempt**" and "**disgust**" - are often played upon, either to make a person do something or to stop a person from doing something. A combination of anger, contempt and disgust can, however, lead to acts of hate and violence. In particular, feelings of contempt and disgust are often used to influence people to distance themselves from others or from a cause.
- Social emotions such as "**pride**," "**guilt**" and "**shame**" are used to influence people to conform to social norms. They are invoked by appealing to our sense of community and our wish to belong to a social network. Studies indicate that the anticipation of pride can be a stronger influencer than the anticipation of negative emotions, such as shame. Shame can be used to make people feel small and to keep them from developing themselves. Guilt can be used to promote behavioral changes and to stimulate empathy and the willingness to show compassion.

- "**Sadness**," "**regret**" and "**hopefulness**," are often leveraged by influencers through forecasting new realities. We are all familiar with the sales pitch "act now," with the implicit suggestion that if we do not act now, we will regret it in the future. Influence that elicits hope is also a strong motivator, as it counteracts feelings of sadness, anxiety and fear. The expression or suggestion of sadness can be effective in motivating a sympathetic response.
- "**Surprise**" helps to attract people's attention, so that they abandon other activities and focus on what the influencer has to say.

Attempts to shape perspectives are operationalized not only by influencing affective mental states, but also by influencing the more epistemic mental states through the way we frame our messages. Let us take a look at some common linguistic tactics:

- "**Self-referencing**," which refers to a technique whereby the influencer uses experiential instructions such as "*Believe me, I promise you things will be better if ...*" or "*Imagine yourself in a situation where ... .*" This technique can lead us to project ourselves into possible future realities and experience associated mental states.
- "**Rhetorical questions**," whereby the influencer uses statements such as "*Don't you want to be a success in life?*" or "*What have they ever done to help us?*" Questions of this nature are most persuasive with people who already share the same mental state of desire or belief, and can be used to affirm and strengthen these mental states.
- "**Vivid language use**," which is a technique used to attract attention by making a message emotionally interesting, image provoking and memorable. This technique taps into our basic and affective mentalizing faculties, which are involved in the detection of affective contagion and the simulation of affective sensations associated with the imagery. In particular, vivid language is used to shape our mental states of desire and belief through their affective components.

- "**Gain/loss framing**," which is a technique whereby the influencer phrases a statement that describes a choice or outcome in terms of its positive (gain) or negative (loss) features. This technique arouses visceral reactions and attracts greater attention to the message. Loss frames have greater persuasive power than gain frames, due to our instinctual predisposition to detect and avoid danger. Gain-framed appeals are better used when the influencer does not want us to devote too much thought to the message, but rather to focus on the reward.
- "**Anchoring**," which plays on our natural bias to rely upon the initial information we receive to "anchor" our subsequent judgments or interpretations. Using this technique, the influencer first presents us with information that is designed to orient our perceptions in a certain way, knowing that it will make us less likely to deviate from this anchor point when making a final decision. This technique can lead to feelings of tension and internal conflict, eroding confidence in our own judgment.
- "**Powerful**," "**powerless**," or "**domineering language**," which involves a particular language style used to hijack mental states. Powerful language conveys certainty. It is used by the influencer to communicate in an impressive and compelling way through confident and forceful statements of facts or beliefs. Powerless language, on the other hand, is sometimes used to create goodwill by making a message seem more personal, down to earth, or human, possibly through feigned uncertainty. Domineering language involves a communication style that contains mandatory assertions such as "*You have no choice*" and "*There is no other way*." This strategy is designed to frighten people into submission, though it often backfires and causes the target of the message to challenge the authority of the influencer.

Through our capacity for mentalization, we monitor changes in the mental states of our target of influence and assess whether these changes shape the target's perspective in the intended manner. Mentalization, as we will now explain, can also help us to predict and prepare for the influence tactics that someone else is likely to use on us.

Predicting the Influencer's Tactic Preference

There are many variables that factor into a person's choice of influence tactics. The situational context and the target of influence are two variables that significantly impact the decision-making process. Other variables include habitual or reactive behavior (i.e., behavior based on what seems to have worked in the past). "Influence tactic choice" is also impacted by our psychological makeup. Early studies indicated that a given personality trait does not significantly predict a particular influence tactic. Mischel and Shoda noted in their 1995 article that "abundant evidence has documented that individual differences in social behaviors tend to be surprisingly variable across different situations." These scholars, however, suggested that the failure to find a significant relationship between personality traits and influence tactic choices might be due to the *design* of the research studies. They presented a new approach: "When personality is conceptualized as a stable system that mediates how the individual selects, construes, and processes social information and generates social behaviors, it becomes possible to account simultaneously for both the invariant qualities of the underlying personality and the predictable variability across situations in some of its characteristic behavioral expressions." In other words, according to Mischel and Shoda, personality consists of predictable "if-then" relationships, and therefore *we should not attempt to predict behavior consistency across all situations*. This approach is known as the "cognitive-affective personality (or processing) system."

The consistency upon which we can predict behavior needs to be found in the *way a person processes social information*. The processing of social information is mediated by personality traits that direct attentional focus, and influence the way information is encoded. As previously discussed, personality traits are reflected in the expression of mental states through behavior or narrative sharing. It is at this level that our mentalization efforts enable us to find regularities in the social information processing of others, which in turn can be used to predict or explain their behavior. Let us apply these principles to a concrete situation.

PREDICTABLE IF-THEN RELATIONSHIPS

Imagine two of your friends sitting in the library, next to a group of noisy students. Both of your friends may share the same desire for peace and quiet. Nevertheless, the tactic each one chooses to address the situation, can be quite different depending upon the way they process social information, given their individual personality traits. If one of your friends has an agreeable disposition, and processes the noise-making as *"these people are just having some fun,"* you would probably predict that your agreeable friend will politely ask the students to tone it down a bit. If the other friend is highly conscientious, he might process this behavior as *"these people don't know how to behave in a library,"* and you could reasonably expect your conscientious friend to approach the students, explain the library rules, including the reasons for these rules, and expect them to conform their behavior accordingly. If, however, you also know that your highly agreeable friend has a low internal locus of control (perceiving himself as having little influence on the world around him), then you might predict that he will simply make a half-hearted effort to influence the noisy students, by clearing his throat and smiling politely when they look in his direction. Similarly, if you know that your conscientious friend struggles with social anxiety, then you might predict that this person will be wary of confronting the group, and instead will ask your agreeable friend to explain the library rules to the students.

RESEARCH EXAMPLES

There are few studies that have examined the relationship between "personality traits" and "preferred influence tactics." Lund et al. (2007)

examined this relationship in a work environment in which people are in "hierarchy negotiation" (i.e., the means by which people maintain or improve their status or position relative to others). The influence tactic choices of their research subjects indicated that:

- Individuals *low* in "agreeableness," and individuals *low* in "conscientiousness," were associated with deceptive and manipulative tactics such as deceptive self-promotion, derogation of others, boasting, aggression, use of sex, exclusion of others, or ingratiation with superiors.
- Individuals *high* in "agreeableness" were engaged in friendship-related social networking activities, but made less use of opportunistic social display tactics.
- Individuals *high* in "extraversion" or "surgency" (a personality trait marked by cheerfulness, responsiveness, spontaneity and sociability) were associated with social display and networking tactics, such as helping others, cultivating friendships, displaying positive social characteristics, social participation, attracting the opposite sex, enhancing appearance, displaying athleticism, etc.
- Individuals *high* in "extraversion" or "surgency," in "conscientiousness," or in "openness to new experiences," and individuals *low* in "neuroticism" were associated with industriousness and knowledge tactics, such as displaying knowledge, working hard, advancing professionally, obtaining education or knowledge, organizing and strategizing, assuming leadership, holding one's own, conforming, enlisting aid, impressing others, socializing selectively, etc.

In a 2006 meta-analytic review conducted by Barbuto and Wheeler, it was found that individuals *high* in "internal locus of control" tended to use logic as a preferred influence tactic, probably because they operate from the belief that they can exert control over their social environment, and therefore do not need to use indirect influence tactics.

Kacmar et al. found in their 2004 study that individuals *low* in "self-esteem" are inclined to use other-focused ingratiation as an influence tactic in the workplace. They found the opposite to be true with individuals *high* in "need for power,"

> [t]hat is, individuals with low self-esteem may have a difficult time bragging about themselves, but can easily fall into the subservient role and position [vis-à-vis] others as the center of attention. The significant relationships between need for power and the other-focused ingratiatory behaviors of other-enhancing and favor rendering suggest that individuals with a high need for power may be less inclined to use other-focused tactics.

They also found that shy people tend to use more self-promotion tactics "to draw attention to their work behaviors in an effort to produce positive reactions from others."

In the aforementioned 1992 article by Buss, it was reported that:

- Individuals *high* in "surgency" tended to use coercion and responsibility invocation, while individuals *low* in "surgency" tended to use self-debasement as a tactic.
- Individuals *high* in "agreeableness" tended to use pleasure induction, while individuals *low* in the same trait were inclined to use coercion.
- *Highly* "conscientious" individuals, and those *high* in "openness" (intellect), tended to use reason to influence others.
- Individuals *high* in "emotional instability" (neuroticism) were more likely to use the influence tactic of regression.

In earlier chapters, we introduced you to the Dark Triad personality constructs (i.e., narcissism, psychopathy and machiavellianism). A 2012 study by Jonason and Webster on Dark Triad personalities, concluded that these personality constructs were correlated with unique tactical choices. The researchers noted "that each trait provides for a variety of tactics of social influence, creating a veritable toolbox of means to manipulate others." Jonason and Webster also proposed that Dark Triad personalities may adopt a "protean approach" (alternating between influence tactics) to effect interpersonal influence, as they do not want to be "found out" by the targets of their influence. The study further indicated, however, that these people do not seem to take individual aspects of their target into account in order to select the best influence tactic. This indicates a lack of mentalizing, which is not surprising, as research indicates the disinclination of such individuals to mentalize about others. It is important to keep in mind, however, that this disinclination to mentalize is often more related to *motivation* and not necessarily to mentalization deficiencies (Esperger & Bereczkei, 2012). Members of the Dark Triad personality construct operate from a strong goal-directed disposition, predominantly using their strategic mentalizing abilities, coupled with a low consideration of the consequences that their behaviors have on others (or on their relationships with others). Their strategies seem to be more premeditated. Their use of mentalization mediates their choice of influence tactics. For instance, a 2014 study conducted by Bo et al. found that "the ability to attribute mental states to others mediates the relation between psychopathy and type of aggression. This mediation is facilitated by a specific mentalization profile characterized by the presence of intact cognitive and deficient affective mentalizing capacities." The fact that Dark Triad personalities seem to work from premeditated tactics might make them more predictable in their choice of influence tactics. Jonason and Webster (2012) note "those high on the Dark Triad traits may have a standard-yet-varied toolkit for social influence they deploy on everyone." These researchers further found that:

- Individuals *high* in "machiavellianism" were generally inclined to use the influence tactics of charm, hardball and seduction to manipulate others. Machiavellianism was not associated with the use of pleasure induction or responsibility invocation.
- Individuals *high* in "psychopathy" also used charm, hardball and seduction, though seduction was used predominantly to manipulate

opposite-sex friends. Unlike machiavellians, psychopaths also used coercion. Psychopathy was not associated with the use of the silent treatment and/or pleasure induction tactics.

- Individuals *high* in "narcissism" were inclined to use charm, coercion, debasement, responsibility invocation and social tactics.
- None of the Dark Triad traits were associated with the use of regression.

In addition, Jonason and Webster explain that "it is primarily machiavellianism that accounted for variability in the adoption of numerous tactics of social influence, perhaps because machiavellianism is characterized by an exploitative interpersonal style (citation omitted)." They proposed that "[o]ne might conclude that machiavellianism is particularly strongly correlated with tactics of social influence, whereas psychopathy is not." Could this suggest that individuals high in machiavellianism use their mentalization capacities more readily than individuals high in narcissism or psychopathy? The scarce available data seems to indicate that although the affective mentalizing capacity of machiavellians seems to be below average, their more cognitive strategic mentalizing capacity is not at all substandard (i.e., Repacholi et al., 2003). And, as previously noted, despite having below average affective mentalizing abilities, given the right motivation, machiavellians are quite capable of taking affective mental states into account. Having discussed the influence tactics that different people use, we will now examine the influenceability of people.

The Target of Influence

Proficiency in influencing others does not necessarily translate into skillful detection and resistance of the unwanted influence of others. As with influence tactic choices, our ability to detect and resist social influence is mediated by a broad range of variables, such as the influence tactic used, the influencer, our current state of mind, our temperament and personality traits, our past experiences, situational factors, etc. We are all susceptible to social influence. Some people, however, seem to be more susceptible to it than others. This can be explained by differences between people in their psychological makeup. In addition, some people who might not seem to be particularly susceptible to social influence, might still be vulnerable to certain specific influence tactics. Let us take a look at research on the relationship between psychological dispositions and influenceability, starting with intrapersonal dispositions.

INTRAPERSONAL DISPOSITIONS

In general, people who lack a well-defined identity, those who are low in self-efficacy and self-esteem, and those who have an external locus of control tend to be more influenceable. These intrapersonal dispositions are related to weak personal boundaries and a low sense of self-determination. In particular, tactics that increase feelings of insecurity and uncertainty tend to yield compliance by these individuals.

With regard to self-consciousness, Froming and Carver found in a 1981 study that individuals who were *high* in "private self-consciousness" (the degree to which people are conscious about their own mental states and covert self-aspects) are less susceptible to social influence than people who are *high* in "public self-consciousness" (the degree to which people are conscious about external aspects of themselves - physical appearance and behavior that can be observed by others). The researchers suggested that "persons high in public self-consciousness are not motivated by a desire to please others, but may be motivated by a desire to 'get along' socially."

Differences from one person to the next in "self-monitoring" habits (noting and adjusting one's behavior in response to situational demands) correlate with variations in their responses to different persuasion tactics. People high in self-monitoring tend to tailor their behavior to the particular circumstances, while people low in self-monitoring are more likely to follow their internal feelings. Evans and Clark found in their 2012 study that people *high* in "self-monitoring" were more easily persuaded by attractive people, while people *low* in "self-monitoring" were more easily persuaded by experts. Self-monitoring, as part of comprehensive intrapersonal mentalizing, can actually increase our awareness of, and resistance to, unwanted influence. Studies also reveal gender difference with regard to susceptibility to different influence tactics. Guadagno and Cialdini (2002), for instance, show that men are more easily persuaded by rational influence tactics in email communications. Women, on the other hand, are more easily influenced by persuasion in person, and by social cues in general.

Although the majority of the studies do not find evidence that people *high* in "extraversion" are more susceptible to one tactic over another, Hirsh et al. found in their 2012 study on persuasive messages, that when messages were framed so that they appealed to excitement and social rewards, extraverts were more easily persuaded. Bowers (1963) found that extroverts, in comparison to introverts, changed their minds more readily in favor of a certain concept when a rational influence tactic was used. Janis (1954) found that individuals with personality characteristics related to the personality trait of agreeableness were associated with compliance. Further, individuals *high* in "agreeableness" seemed to be especially susceptible to reciprocal influence tactics. When reciprocity was perceived as a social norm, these individuals felt obligated to yield to others. In addition, Hirsh et al. (2012) found messages that appealed to family and community were particularly influential with highly agreeable people.

Individuals *high* in "interpersonal dependency" have a high degree of suggestibility, conformity and compliance. Bornstein (1992) noted that:

> First, dependency is associated with a general tendency to be influenced by the opinions of others, to yield to others in interpersonal transactions, and to comply with others' expectations and demands. However, when placed in a position in which they must choose between pleasing a peer or pleasing a figure of authority, the dependent person will typically opt for pleasing the authority figure.

Likewise, people with an authoritarian disposition yield more readily to the dictates of authority figures. At odds with the view they have of themselves as strong leaders, insecurity and low self-esteem underlie the authoritarian personality (Larsen & Schwendiman, 1969).

It should come as no surprise that Dark Triad personalities score *low* on "compliance." Paradoxically, however, secondary psychopathy is associated with *high* "impulsivity" (Poythress et al., 2011), which has been tentatively linked to higher levels of compliance (Ray & Jones, 2012). Yildirim (2016) explains that,

> [t]he core pathology in primary psychopathy [is] a deficiency of emotion, caused largely by genetic factors, and the core pathology in secondary psychopathy [is] a disturbance of emotion, caused mainly by destructive environmental influences on emotional and moral development.

Attachment styles also mediate the level of suggestibility. Drake found in her 2010 study that people with a fearful avoidant attachment style comply more readily to negative feedback in interrogative interviews. Drake explains that "[c]ompliance may have developed as a coping method in the face of more intensely negative events."

AFFECTIVE DISPOSITIONS

Researchers have also studied the relationship between affective dispositions and persuasibility. For instance, neuroticism, a personality trait commonly found in individuals *high* in "attachment anxiety" and "avoidance," is strongly associated with susceptibility to influence. Gudjonsson et al. found in their 2004 study that the neurotic person's level of introversion moderated this relationship. Individuals *high* in both "neuroticism" and "introversion" are the most compliant. A general sense of insecurity may underlie or contribute to this tendency toward susceptibility to influence. People who struggle with depression are more easily persuaded when they think that the influencer can alleviate the cause of their suffering.

Positive affective states of the influence target can diminish the level at which influence messages are processed. Happy people tend to rely more on peripheral cues than on central information processing. The impact of positive affects, however, depends on aspects such as confidence in one's own thinking, and on the quality of the arguments in a message (Briñol et al., 2007).

Individuals *high* in "social anxiousness," "shyness" and "embarrassability," and those prone to "shame" or "guilt," are associated with high compliance, especially in regard to influence tactics such as responsibility invocation, reciprocity and social comparison.

Individuals *high* in "hostility" and prone to "anger" are associated with low impulse control, which makes them more vulnerable to certain influence tactics, particularly those that play on the individual's angry and hostile disposition. In other respects, however, these individuals tend to score *low* on "susceptibility to social influence."

People who experience affects more intensely have an increased susceptibility to influence, as influencers often resort to emotional appeals. Intense emotions can, however, turn such influence targets away if they find the emotional appeal too overwhelming.

COGNITIVE DISPOSITIONS

When we move away from affective dispositions to cognitive dispositions, intelligence level, as classically assessed, is significantly associated with suggestibility in the sense that highly intelligent people are more resistant to influence than people of low intelligence. People of high intelligence tend to grasp a message and its underlying meaning more quickly, and engage in more extensive critical thinking. Many influence tactics are, however, cleverly designed to bypass careful systematic processing of information. Evidence also exists that highly intelligent people may nevertheless be vulnerable to influence tactics, since their cognitive capacity allows them to rationalize faulty decisions, a process called "motivated reasoning." In a sense, this can be seen as a form of confirmation bias. Motivated reasoning flows from an unconscious bias toward decisions that conform to something a person already knows, even in the face of evidence to the contrary. Additionally, some intelligent people prefer to base their decisions on intuition rather than reflective, analytical thinking. A rational thinking style is commonly assessed with an instrument known as the "cognitive reflection test" (CRT) (Frederick, 2005), which measures the tendency to override an incorrect initial response, and to engage in reflective reasoning that leads to the correct response. People who score poorly on the CRT tend to be more susceptible to fake news, conspiracy theories and paranormal thinking (Pennycook & Rand, 2019). People with a *high* "need for cognition" (the motivation to engage in effortful cognitive activities) have a preference for careful and systematic processing of information. These individuals are less susceptible to misinformation, since they engage more naturally in discrepancy detection (Leding & Antonio, 2019).

The disposition toward a "need for cognitive closure" is also associated with the level of cognitive scrutiny. People *high* in this personality trait desire a clear conclusion (closure) as quickly as possible (urgency tendency), and they prefer to adhere to their initial conclusion, as they have an aversion toward ambiguity (permanence tendency) (Kruglanski et al., 1996). These individuals are prone to bias, forming conclusions on the basis of early judgmental cues, and dispensing with critical analysis. This tendency to process information in a heuristic manner is mediated by increasing the stakes of an inaccurate conclusion.

Individuals having a disposition toward "richness of fantasy" tend to be more receptive to persuasive communications (Janis & Field, 1959). Vivid imagination might strengthen the ability for mental time travel, allowing the projection of such a person into a possible future reality with the anticipation of potential rewards or punishments that are suggested by the influencer.

The "openness to experience" personality trait is associated with a *low* preference for consistency, which makes individuals having this disposition more persuasible. They tend to place more value on new stimuli than on earlier choices and commitments (Cialdini et al., 1995). Messages that appeal to creativity and intellectual stimulation can be very influential with these people (Hirsh et al., 2012). On the other hand, such people have an inquisitive way of processing information that might protect them from mindless acquiescence with influence.

MOTIVATIONAL DISPOSITION

Motivational dispositions can also have an impact on susceptibility to influence. One such motivational disposition is conscientiousness, which consists of such traits as detail-orientedness, diligence and goal-directedness. People *high* in "conscientiousness" set goals and work toward them in an organized fashion. These people are *low* in "impulsiveness" and *high* in "emotional stability" (DeYoung et al., 2002). Conscientiousness correlates positively with rule compliance, obedience and conventional integrity. In a study based on the Milgram experiments (Bègue et al., 2014), conscientiousness and agreeableness were associated with the willingness to administer high-intensity electric shocks to a victim. Conscientious people, owing largely to their reliance on conformity, tend to be vulnerable to social influence, preferring to act in a socially desirable way. They have a lower tendency for exploration and reconceptualization, and they tend to be low in impulsivity. On the other hand, these personality characteristics make them less susceptive to influential tactics that require them to step away from earlier commitments, to adjust their initial plans, or to adapt to new behaviors. Messages that appeal to effectiveness and goal pursuit are influential with people who score *high* on "conscientiousness" (Hirsh et al., 2012).

Finally, people can differ significantly in the fundamental motives upon which they base important life decisions. There are, for instance, individuals with a general motivational disposition for achieving success, for belonging and affiliating, for power and material gain, etc. These fundamental motives make people more vulnerable to influence tactics that are congruent with their objectives. To illustrate, people who are materialistic more easily fall for con artist tactics that promise high returns.

TEMPORARY MENTAL STATES AND CONTEXT

As we have seen, certain dispositional characteristics can make a person more susceptible to influence, while others increase their resistance to influence. These dispositional characteristics can operate within the same person on various different levels (intrapersonal, interpersonal, affective, cognitive, motivational). For instance, an intelligent but empathetic person may identify an influence tactic as specious, but still yield to it based on its emotional appeal. Even dispositional characteristics operating at the same level (e.g., need for cognition, need for cognitive closure) can work at cross purposes. Beyond dispositional factors, we need to remember that temporary mental states, such as fatigue and a sense of urgency, can make us more vulnerable to influence tactics. Furthermore, the specific tactic used by the influencer mediates the susceptibility of people to social influence. Likewise, contextual aspects often play a significant role in determining the susceptibility of a person to influence tactics. For instance, in a group setting, we may be more influenced by the response of others to a manipulation tactic than to the tactic itself. Additionally, the relationship between influencer and target (professional, familial, etc.) can impact susceptibility to influence. A friend or family member might be more influential than a stranger, and we may yield more readily to an authority figure, such as a teacher or manager, than to a peer. Finally, some people are simply master manipulators, making it difficult for anyone, under any circumstances, to resist their influence.

Resisting Unwanted Influence

Resisting relentless attempts by advertisers, social media, family, friends or colleagues, to influence is not easy for anyone. As we have seen, simply being smart is not a guarantee against falling prey to the manipulative influence of others. Despite published research and other guidance on methods of detecting and resisting misleading influence tactics, it seems as though we will always remain vulnerable to manipulative influence techniques. One theory explains how our state of mind at any given time impacts our susceptibility to influence. Guadagno (2017) describes the "mindlessness hypothesis," as a mechanism underlying the effectiveness of compliance tactics. She explains that "[compliance tactics] work best under situations in which an influence target uses heuristics rather than deep thought to guide decision-making." Guadagno posits that "[t]hose under cognitive load engage more in peripheral processing of the message. When people have full access to their attentional resources, they can centrally process a message." "Cognitive load" refers to the percentage of a person's working memory capacity that is being used at any given time. When our processing capacity is being taxed, we tend to more readily succumb to the influence tactic.

Influence attempts by those using manipulation tactics start with finding a vulnerability through mentalization, or through pseudomentalization (such as that used by psychics). This can be a particular sensitivity, an insecurity, a feeling of inadequacy, or a sense that we are missing out on something. Paradoxically, it is our effort to hide these vulnerabilities that makes us more vulnerable. We unwittingly attract more attention to our weak spots, inviting the influencer to exploit them. When confronted with influence tactics that target our vulnerabilities, we narrow our intrapersonal mentalizing efforts to the point that they become self-conscious, rather than self-reflective. Our rational thinking is preempted by a preoccupation with our shortcomings or sensitivities. At the same time, our mentalizing about the influencer is arrested, and the influencer seizes the opportunity to offer a solution that makes us feel good, that relieves our uncomfortable feelings, or that provides us with a false sense of security or control.

One general resistance strategy to unwanted influence is described by the "inoculation theory," developed by social psychologist William J. McGuire (McGuire, 1961). This theory explains how we remain true to our existing attitudes and beliefs in the face of attempts to change them. Inoculation is a technique developed to strengthen existing attitudes and beliefs, while building resistance to future counterarguments. The influence inoculation process is analogous to the medical inoculation process from which it draws its name. Traditional methods of medical inoculation worked by introducing a weakened form of a virus into an organism - one that would trigger the organism's production of antibodies, but not overwhelm the organism's resistance. Influence inoculation uses the same approach. We prepare ourselves in advance by considering weakened arguments that a potential influencer might use to challenge beliefs that we hold about someone, something or a situation. The threat of the challenge to our beliefs prompts us to develop counterarguments, which provide us with a form of resistance against stronger persuasive messages or arguments advanced by the influencer. The effect of an inoculation can persist for weeks or even months. In reality, however, it isn't feasible to inoculate ourselves against every situation that we might encounter in life. When it comes to identifying and assessing influence attempts, real-time mentalization provides us with a better opportunity to accurately detect influence tactics and respond to them in an appropriate way.

Resistance to unwanted influence can be evaluated from two perspectives:

1. The "**outcome**" (whether or not we have yielded to the influence tactic); and
2. The "**influence process**" (how we came to resist or yield to the influence tactic).

An examination of the influence process highlights the role of mentalization in detecting and resisting unwanted influence. Mentalization involves inferring the mental states of others through keen observations of their verbal and nonverbal behavior, while simultaneously monitoring our own mental states. Interpersonal mentalizing enables us to establish a behavioral baseline for others. Once we have established this baseline, we can detect changes in behavior that reveal fluctuations in the other's mental states. We need to look for signals and cues such as:

- Variations in behavioral styles with different people, in different situations, or in the course of the same situation. While this type of social differentiation is normal to a certain extent, it is noteworthy when applied in an extreme fashion (e.g., being extremely polite to one person and completely rude to another).
- Fluctuation between a relaxed composure and agitation or heightened arousal, especially in response to requests for additional information or clarification. This could signify that the influencer simply does not possess the requested information, but it could also point to attempts to deceive or manipulate.
- Abandonment by the influencer of his or her personal values and motivational drives in favor of appeals to our own, in an attempt to convince us of something.
- Attempts to characterize relational status in a way that is incongruent with the situation or the existing relationship (e.g., someone pretending to be your best friend when they just met you).
- Use of a form of pseudomentalization (pretending to know how we feel, what we desire, or what we are thinking).

Likewise, intrapersonal mentalizing is necessary to establish an experiential baseline for ourselves, relative to which we can detect changes within ourselves such as:

- Sensing a heightened state of alertness. When we are being manipulated, our survival instinct will be activated to produce an affective reaction.
- Sensing confusion and insecurity. An influencer may try to create "cognitive dissonance," a mental state of conflicting thoughts, beliefs, or attitudes, especially relating to behavioral decisions and attitude changes. Alternatively, the influencer may attempt to make us doubt our own perceptions. "Gaslighting," for instance, is a tactic whereby a person or entity constructs alternative versions of reality in order to make us question our own sense of reality and sanity.

- Questioning our own behavior or beliefs. We may entertain thoughts such as *"I never thought I would do or say something like that,"* or *"Why am I defending a position that I don't even agree with myself?"*
- Sensing feelings of low self-esteem. An influencer may try to make us feel inadequate, so that we will be more likely to surrender our power or rights.
- Sensing moral emotions. For instance, an influencer may try to make us feel guilty for failing to comply with a request.
- Sensing reactance. "Reactance" refers to an unpleasant motivational arousal to offers, people, rules, or regulations that threaten behavioral freedom of choice.

The detection of interoceptive sensations and changes in our affective and cognitive mental states, especially those that we associate with our "weak spots," are tell-tale signs that we may be the target of unwanted influence. Let us look at different ways that mentalization can help us increase our influential power.

Increasing Influential Power Through Mentalization

Strategic mentalizing helps to lay the groundwork for a robust foundation of influential power. Influential power is needed both for exercising influence, and for resisting unwanted influence. Influential power derives from various sources:

- "**Personal power**:" Intrapersonal mentalizing fosters a type of power that has as its principal aim self-realization (mastery of self). Personal power is based on personal qualities such as a high level of self-regulation and self-efficacy, and a well-formed self-identity, with clear personal boundaries. People who possess personal power tend to be more at ease with others, more supportive of others, and display a healthy level of empathy and compassion. They tend to stay true to their own beliefs and convictions, and are therefore better influencers when promoting these beliefs and convictions. At the same time, and for many of the same reasons, they are more resistant to influence by others.

- "**Informational power**:" Strategic mentalizing, supported by basic and affective mentalizing, helps us to collect and process social information. The predictive and explanatory value of this information increases our power to influence social outcomes, and to detect unwanted influence at an early stage.
- "**Goal-directed focus**:" Strategic mentalizing helps us to maintain a consistent and focused course in our cooperative and competitive endeavors, keeping us on track notwithstanding the attempts of others to move us in a different direction.
- "**Referent power**:" This power is associated with the qualities of charisma, integrity and self-assuredness. It is widely considered to be the most valuable type of power. People who use their mentalization competencies to demonstrate mastery and control over their environment have a natural ability to attract, persuade and inspire others. The properties of this power also ward off unwanted influence.
- "**Social network**" and "**connection power**:" Strategic mentalizing enables us to connect to, and affiliate with, the right people, and conversely, to keep a safe distance from the wrong people. Connection power derives from an affiliation with people who have a healthy level of influential power, and who are willing to share it with us.
- "**Moral power**:" This is a power resulting from mentalization efforts that reflect healthy and appropriate conduct in our interactions with others. Moral power has the potential to inspire other people to view us as positive role models.

Thus, the power to influence others and to resist unwanted influence is strengthened through strategic mentalizing. Because strategic mentalizing competency correlates positively with our level of influential power, we can gauge our strategic mentalizing competency indirectly by assessing our ability to influence our social environment. Let us take a closer look at how we can assess our strategic mentalizing competency.

Assessing Strategic Mentalizing Competency

The fact that people react in a manner that we predicted, or in a way that we intended is a clear indication that our strategic mentalizing abilities are functioning at a high level. If we are frequently surprised or confused by the behavior of others, if we feel as though we have little or no control over situations, if we are easily taken advantage of, or if we are regularly disappointed with the outcomes of our personal interactions, we could gain great practical benefits from strengthening our strategic mentalizing competencies. Mentalization effectiveness is also measurable by the influence we have on other people, and by how well we detect and resist the unhealthy influence of others. Good strategic mentalizing manifests itself in favorable outcomes in cooperative and competitive social interactions.

We can assess the efficacy of our strategic mentalizing efforts in answers to such questions as:

How accurate are my predictions of, or explanations for, the behavior of others?
Do I make good use of these predictions and explanations in my dealings with others?
Do my influence tactics produce the desired outcomes?
Am I successful in recognizing and resisting the unhealthy influence of others?

We validate our strategic mentalizing competencies in two ways:

- Through the practice of forward-chaining in predicting the behavior of others. We could, for instance, imagine one scenario that is likely to unfold if we successfully shape a person's perspective, and one that is likely to occur if we do not try to influence their perspective. The more accurate our predictions, the more confident we can be in our mentalization competencies.
- Through the practice of backward-chaining. This entails explaining a situation based upon a critical evaluation of the most plausible scenarios, guided by the perspectives of the various people involved. A high degree of accuracy in our explanations would indicate highly developed strategic mentalizing competencies. Moreover, accurate explanations of past behavior are a valuable information resource for accurate predictions of future behavior. As the saying goes, *"The best predictor of future behavior is past behavior."*

Sharpening Perspective Shaping Competencies: Advantages, Impediments and Avenues for Enhancement

ADVANTAGES

Let us explore how well-developed perspective shaping competencies can yield benefits on different levels. Intrapersonally, by examining the outcomes of our influence efforts *we gain insight into the efficacy of our strategic mentalizing efforts.* Through backward-chaining we can evaluate whether our chosen influence tactics have achieved their intended results. Our mentalization effectiveness is also measured by how well we detect and resist the unhealthy influence of others. Our track record of success in wielding influential power provides a benchmark for assessing our mentalization competence. Conversely, strategic mentalizing helps us to strengthen our influential power, which in turn increases our sense of self-efficacy and self-esteem, and our overall sense of well-being.

Interpersonally, strategic mentalizing *helps us to select the right influence tactics to shape the perspectives of others.* Strategic mentalizing also helps us to adjust our influence strategies if we perceive unintended changes or intransigence in the mental states of others. Additionally, strategic mentalizing *helps us to predict the influence tactics that others are likely to use on us* so that we can "inoculate" ourselves against their efforts. Moreover, our capacity to alternate between intrapersonal and interpersonal mentalizing in real-time *helps us to quickly detect and appropriately respond to the influence tactics of others.* Properly applied influence tactics, guided by sound mentalization efforts, can pay dividends in both cooperative and competitive environments.

Extrapersonally, mentalization can indirectly *bolster influential power to shape the perspective of a larger group and help us to resist unwanted group influence.* Mentalization keeps us focused on our own values and goals, something that is becoming increasingly difficult in the face of external influences presented via the World Wide Web and social media. Imagine what Edward Bernays, "the Father of Spin," could have done with access to these communication tools!

IMPEDIMENTS

Let us examine some of the impediments to perspective shaping. Intrapersonally, research has indicated that *people who view themselves as self-confident, self-determinant and highly competent, tend to be less vigilant of, and therefore more susceptible to, unwanted influence.* While it might be assumed that their self-view would make them less susceptible to influence, in fact, it can also create a false sense of security that makes them less inclined to mentalize and to process influence messages systematically.

Interpersonally, we need to remember that *having a higher status can diminish our mentalization efforts with regard to people whom we perceive as having a lower status.* The resulting "mindblindness" can lead to missed opportunities to choose the best tactics to influence others, or to identify and resist the influence tactics of others.

Extrapersonally, *the constitution of a group can significantly impede our ability to choose the most appropriate influence tactic, or to resist unwanted group influence.* Strategic mentalizing about larger groups can be difficult, as it requires consideration of many different people having potentially diverse sociocultural and economic backgrounds. Influencing a group, or resisting unwanted group influence, is more difficult where there is a great disparity in influential power between the group and the individual. We also tend to view a larger group as having a single collective mind, ignoring the contributing mental states of its various constituent members.

AVENUES FOR ENHANCEMENT

In this chapter, we explored the relationship between strategic mentalizing and influential power. Strategic mentalizing competency correlates positively with our level of influential power. Therefore, we can gauge our mentalization competencies indirectly through assessing the following:

- The accuracy of our predictions or explanations regarding influence behavior.
- The effectiveness of our influence tactics.
- The efficacy of our efforts to recognize and resist unwanted influence of others.

Additionally, we have discussed how well-developed strategic mentalizing can significantly increase our influential power, both to persuade others and to resist the unwanted influence of others. Our perspective shaping competencies are enhanced by mentalizing at other levels as well. Affective mentalizing plays an important role in exerting or resisting influence. It helps us to guard against affective reactions (both our own and those of others) that could disrupt or overwhelm the influence process. Additionally, it helps us to stay emotionally grounded in the face of the manipulative, coercive, or deceptive influence attempts of others. At a fundamental level, basic mentalizing makes us aware of the dynamic impact of nonverbal behavior on the exertion of, or resistance to, influential power.

ETHICAL CONSIDERATIONS

We conclude this chapter by taking a moment to examine the ethical aspects of exerting influential power. Determining whether an exercise of influential power is consistent with sound ethical practices depends on answers to such questions as:

> *What is the motivation behind the attempted influence?*
> *Are the influence tactics appropriate or warranted?*
> *Does the influence target have the power to resist?*

Finding accurate answers to these questions depends, to a large extent, on our capacity to mentalize. Mentalization is the most powerful social tool that we have at our disposal to exert influential power over others. If not guided by ethical practices, mentalization can be used for less than honorable purposes. In the introductory section of this book, we introduced you to a code of conduct governing mentalization. In the previous chapter, we reiterated two ethical principles that are relevant to perspective gaining. We would like to emphasize three additional principles from the code of conduct that are most relevant to perspective shaping:

Principle 1, which stresses that:

> We must remain mindful of the influence and the potential consequences that mentalization can have on individuals and groups with whom we deal, and avoid misuse or abuse at all times.

Principle 3, which advocates that:

> Our mentalizing efforts should not be done in a way that is viewed by others as misleading, exploitative, or intentionally pernicious.

Principle 5, which asserts that:

> Proper mentalization practices should reflect sensitivity to diversity concerns related to such factors as race, ethnicity, gender, religious beliefs, physical or mental disability and socioeconomic status.

SECTION SUMMARY

We have now come to the end of this section on strategic mentalizing, the highest and most cognitive level of mentalization. We have seen that strategic mentalizing enables us to infer the more epistemic mental states, largely inferred through verbal information sharing, in order to form increasingly rational models of what is going on in the minds of others. It entails the use of theory of mind reasoning to either enhance affiliation and cooperation, or to distance ourselves from others and to gain a competitive advantage. It is through the iterative and cyclical processes involving basic, affective and strategic mentalizing, that we advance from common-sense inferences to more critical reasoning based on psychological and sociological knowledge and understanding.

This section was comprised of four chapters. In the first chapter, *Motivation to Mentalize Strategically,* we explored how intrapersonal, interpersonal and extrapersonal factors influence our motivation to strategically mentalize. In the second chapter, *Content Extraction,* we focused on the type of information we look for when we strategically mentalize. In the third chapter, *Perspective Gaining and Shifting,* we examined how we use strategic mentalizing competencies to gain access to the perspectives of others, and to contrast these perspectives with our own, an ability known as perspective shifting. In this chapter, *Perspective Shaping*, we discussed how strategic mentalizing strengthens our power to influence others and to resist the unwanted influence of others.

This brings us to the fifth and final section of the book *Mastering Mentalization* where we will present a self-directed learning model for mastering mentalization.

References

American Psychological Association. (n.d.). Exemplification. In *APA dictionary of psychology*. Retrieved July 17, 2022, from https://dictionary.apa.org/exemplification

American Psychological Association. (n.d.). Self-presentation. In *APA dictionary of psychology*. Retrieved July 17, 2022, from https://dictionary.apa.org/self-presentation

American Psychological Association. (n.d.). Self-promotion. In *APA dictionary of psychology*. Retrieved July 17, 2022, from https://dictionary.apa.org/self-promotion

American Psychological Association. (n.d.). Social comparison theory. In *APA dictionary of psychology*. Retrieved July 17, 2022, from https://dictionary.apa.org/social-comparison-theory

American Psychological Association. (n.d.). Supplication. In *APA dictionary of psychology*. Retrieved July 17, 2022, from https://dictionary.apa.org/supplication

Barbuto, J. E., Jr., & Wheeler, D. W. (2006). Scale Development and Construct Clarification of Servant Leadership. *Group & Organization Management, 31*(3), 300–326. https://doi.org/10.1177/1059601106287091

Bègue, L., Beauvois, J.-L., Courbet, D., Oberlé, D., Lepage, J., & Duke, A. A. (2014). Personality Predicts Obedience in a Milgram Paradigm. *Journal of Personality, 83(3), 299–306.* doi:10.1111/jopy.12104

Bo, S., Abu-Akel, A., Kongerslev, M., Haahr, U. H., & Bateman, A. (2014). Mentalizing mediates the relationship between psychopathy and type of aggression in schizophrenia. *Journal of Nervous and Mental Disease, 202*(1), 55–63. https://doi.org/10.1097/NMD.0000000000000067

Bornstein, R. F. (1992). The dependent personality: Developmental, social, and clinical perspectives. *Psychological Bulletin*, 112(1), 3-23. https://doi.org/10.1037/0033-2909.112.1.3

Bowers, J. W. (1963). Language intensity, social introversion, and attitude change. *Speech Monographs*, 30, 345-352. https://doi.org/10.1080/03637756309375380

Briñol, P., Petty, R. E., & Barden, J. (2007). Happiness versus sadness as a determinant of thought confidence in persuasion: A self-validation analysis. *Journal of Personality and Social Psychology, 93*(5), 711–727. doi:10.1037/0022-3514.93.5.711

Buss, D. M., Gomes, M., Higgins, D. S., & Lauterbach, K. (1987). Tactics of manipulation. *Journal of Personality and Social Psychology, 52*(6), 1219–1229. doi: 10.1037/0022-3514.52.6.1219

Buss, D. M. (1992). Manipulation in close relationships: Five personality factors in interactional context. *Journal of Personality, 60*(2), 477–499. https://doi.org/10.1111/j.1467-6494.1992.tb00981.x

Carli, L. L. (2017). *Social influence and gender*. In S. Harkins, K. D. Williams & J. Burger, (Eds.), *The Oxford handbook of social influence*. Oxford University Press.

Cialdini, R. B. (2009). *Influence: Science and practice* (5th ed.). Allyn & Bacon.

Cialdini, R. B. (2016). *Pre-Suasion: A Revolutionary Way to Influence and Persuade*. Simon and Schuster.

Cialdini, R. B., Trost, M. R., & Newsom, J. T. (1995). Preference for consistency: The development of a valid measure and the discovery of surprising behavioral implications. *Journal of Personality and Social Psychology, 69*(2), 318–328. https://doi.org/10.1037/0022-3514.69.2.318

Drake, K. E. (2010). The psychology of interrogative suggestibility: A vulnerability during interview. *Personality and Individual Differences, 49*(7), 683–688. doi:10.1016/j.paid.2010.06.005

DeYoung, C. G., Peterson, J. B., & Higgins, D. M. (2002). Higher-order factors of the Big Five predict conformity: Are there neuroses of health? *Personality and Individual Differences, 33*(4), 533–552. https://doi.org/10.1016/S0191-8869(01)00171-4

Esperger, Z., & Bereczkei, T. (2012). Machiavellianism and spontaneous mentalization: One step ahead of others. *European Journal of Personality, 26*(6), 580–587. https://doi.org/10.1002/per.859

Evans, A. T., & Clark, J. K. (2012). Source characteristics and persuasion: The role of self-monitoring in self-validation. *Journal of Experimental Social Psychology, 48*(1), 383–386. https://doi.org/10.1016/j.jesp.2011.07.002

Frederick, S. (2005). Cognitive Reflection and Decision Making. *Journal of Economic Perspectives, 19*(4), 25–42. doi:10.1257/089533005775196732

Froming, W. J., & Carver, C. S. (1981). Divergent influences of private and public self-consciousness in a compliance paradigm. *Journal of Research in Personality, 15*(2), 159–171. https://doi.org/10.1016/0092-6566(81)90015-5

Guadagno, R. E. (2017). *Compliance: A classic and contemporary review*. In S. Harkins, K. D. Williams & J. Burger, (Eds.), *The Oxford handbook of social influence*. Oxford University Press.

Guadagno, R. E., & Cialdini, R. B. (2002). Online persuasion: An examination of gender differences in computer-mediated interpersonal influence. *Group Dynamics: Theory, Research, and Practice, 6*(1), 38–51. https://doi.org/10.1037/1089-2699.6.1.38

Gudjonsson, G. H., Sigurdsson, J. F., Bragason, O. O., Einarsson, E., & Valdimarsdottir, E. B. (2004). Compliance and personality: the vulnerability of the unstable introvert. *European Journal of Personality, 18*(5), 435–443. doi:10.1002/per.514

Hales, H. H., Ren, D., & Williams, K. D. (2017). Protect, correct, and eject: Ostracism as a social influence tool. In S. Harkins, K. D. Williams & J. Burger, (Eds.), *The Oxford handbook of social influence*. Oxford University Press.

Harkins, S., Williams, K. D., & Burger, J. (Eds.) (2017). *The Oxford handbook of social influence*. Oxford University Press.

Hirsh, J. B., Kang, S. K., & Bodenhausen, G. V. (2012). Personalized persuasion: Tailoring persuasive appeals to recipients' personality traits. *Psychological Science, 23*(6), 578–581. https://doi.org/10.1177/0956797611436349

Janis, I. L. (1954). Personality correlates of susceptibility to persuasion. *Journal of Personality, 22*, 504–518. https://doi.org/10.1111/j.1467-6494.1954.tb01870.x

Janis, I. L., & Field, P. B. (1959). *Sex differences and personality factors related to persuasibility*. In C. I. Hovland & I. L. Janis (Eds.), *Personality and persuasibility* (pp. 62-63). New Haven, CT: Yale University Press.

Jonason, P. K., & Webster, G. D. (2012). A protean approach to social influence: Dark Triad personalities and social influence tactics. *Personality and Individual Differences, 52*(4), 521–526. doi:10.1016/j.paid.2011.11.023

Milgram, S. (1963). Behavioral study of obedience. *Journal of abnormal and social psychology, 67*, 371-378. https://doi.org/10.1037/h0040525

Mischel W., & Shoda, Y. (1995). A cognitive-affective system theory of personality: reconceptualizing situations, dispositions, dynamics, and invariance in personality structure. *Psychological Review, 102*(2), 246-68. doi: 10.1037/0033-295x.102.2.246.

Kacmar, K. M., Carlson, D. S., & Bratton, V. K. (2004). Situational and dispositional factors as antecedents of ingratiatory behaviors in organizational settings. *Journal of Vocational Behavior, 65*(2), 309–331. https://doi.org/10.1016/j.jvb.2003.09.002

Kruglanski, A. W., & Webster, D. M. (1996). Motivated closing of the mind: "Seizing" and "freezing." *Psychological Review, 103*(2), 263–283. doi:10.1037/0033-295x.103.2.263

Larsen, K. S., & Schwendiman, G. (1969). Authoritarianism, self esteem and insecurity. *Psychological Reports* 25(1):229-30. doi:10.2466/pr0.1969.25.1.229

Leding, J. K., & Antonio, L. (2019). Need for cognition and discrepancy detection in the misinformation effect. *Journal of Cognitive Psychology, 31*(4), 409–415. doi:10.1080/20445911.2019.1626400

Lund, O. C. H., Tamnes, C. K., Moestue, C., Buss, D. M., & Vollrath, M. (2007). Tactics of hierarchy negotiation. *Journal of Research in Personality, 41*(1), 25–44. https://doi.org/10.1016/j.jrp.2006.01.002

McGuire, W. J. (1961). "Resistance to persuasion conferred by active and passive prior refutation of same and alternative counterarguments". *Journal of Abnormal Psychology*. 63 (2): 326–332. doi:10.1037/h0048344.Poythress, N.

G., & Hall, J. R. (2011). Psychopathy and impulsivity reconsidered. *Aggression and Violent Behavior, 16*(2), 120–134. doi:10.1016/j.avb.2011.02.003

Pennycook, G., & Rand, D. G. (2019). Who falls for fake news? The roles of bullshit receptivity, overclaiming, familiarity, and analytic thinking. Journal of Personality. doi:10.1111/jopy.12476

Ray, J. V., & Jones, S. (2012). Examining the relationship between self-reported compliance and psychopathic personality traits. *Personality and Individual Differences, 52*(2), 190–194. doi:10.1016/j.paid.2011.10.011

Repacholi, B., Slaughter, V., Pritchard, M., & Gibbs, V. (2003). *Theory of mind, Machiavellianism, and social functioning in childhood.* In B. Repacholi & V. Slaughter (Eds.), *Macquarie monographs in cognitive science. Individual differences in theory of mind: Implications for typical and atypical development* (p. 67–97). Psychology Press.

Yildirim, B. O. (2016). A treatise on secondary psychopathy: Psychobiological pathways to severe antisociality. *Aggression and Violent Behavior, 31,* 165–185. doi:10.1016/j.avb.2016.09.004

SECTION V.

MASTERING MENTALIZATION

To Understand and Practice

A Metacognitive Learning Approach

In this final section, we provide you with a "self-directed learning model" for mastering mentalization. This model employs a *metacognitive learning approach,* a term which refers to the cognitive processes that humans use to plan, monitor and assess their own learning activities and progress. We view "metacognitive learning" as the most suitable approach for mastering mentalization, because there is no rigid formula for learning these skills: *no two minds work exactly the same way and there is no inherently superior learning style.* Additionally, the self-directed learning model provides you with guidelines for designing your own learning trajectory. Metacognitive learning helps you to gauge your knowledge level and to find, select and practice learning strategies that best fit your learning style, needs and contextual demands.

Metacognition is thinking about the way we think, and often includes a conscious attempt to manage our own thought processes. "Meta" means beyond, and "cognition" refers to the mental processes of acquiring knowledge and understanding through thought, experience and sensory data. Metacognitive learning involves viewing ourselves as both thinker and learner.

Metacognition is a complex concept often subject to misunderstanding. Two common misconceptions worth noting:

1. The first misconception is *that metacognition is the same thing as executive functioning, self-regulation, or theory of mind reasoning.* Metacognition involves thinking about, assessing and enhancing our executive functioning, self-regulation and mentalization capacities. Executive functioning and self-regulation, on the other hand, are the essential building blocks for higher order thinking skills, such as metacognition, critical thinking and attributional complexity. Theory of mind reasoning is one particular form of metacognition. Kuhn (2000) describes theory of mind reasoning as a form of metacognitive knowing - knowledge that mental states exist - which we separate into: "intrapersonal metacognitive knowing," referring to knowledge about one's own mental states; "interpersonal metacognitive knowing," referring to knowledge about the mental states of others; and "extrapersonal metacognitive knowing," referring to group knowledge.
2. The second misconception is closely related to the first. It posits that *when we are good at metacognitive learning, we will thrive in all other cognitive abilities.* Metacognitive learning helps us to become aware of weaknesses in our thinking with regard to our own cognitive abilities, and it is essential for assessing and evaluating our learning progress. Nevertheless, we need to combine this awareness with specific subject matter knowledge and practice to enhance our mentalization competencies, executive functioning and self-regulation.

Schraw and Dennison (1994) divided metacognition into two components: knowledge and regulation. "Metacognitive knowledge" includes:

- "**Declarative**" **knowledge**, which refers to understanding our own level of knowledge about something (in this case, what we know about mentalization). It also includes our level of awareness about what we do not know.
- "**Procedural**" **knowledge**, which refers to understanding of the cognitive strategies that can be applied in furtherance of our knowledge and skills.
- "**Conditional**" **knowledge**, which refers to our strategic understanding of when, where and why we should use declarative and procedural knowledge.

"Metacognitive regulation" includes:

- "**Planning skills**," which can be described as the ability to choose the appropriate metacognitive learning strategies and to allocate the required resources.
- "**Comprehension**" and "**process monitoring skills**," which refer to our ongoing assessment of our application of declarative and procedural knowledge.
- **"Evaluation skills**," which refer to the appraisal of our learning progress and the effectiveness of our learning strategies, including the consideration of new metacognitive learning strategies, as necessary.

Eight Steps to Mastering Mentalization

Research indicates that metacognitive awareness is a powerful predictor of learning. Moreover, metacognitive skills help us to extend what we have learned in one context to another, or from a previous interaction to a new encounter. Learning to master mentalization by using metacognitive skills consists of the following eight steps:

1. Establish a personal mentalization profile to provide a baseline (*What do I already know about mentalizing, and how do I currently use mentalization?*)
2. Identify criteria against which you can judge your learning progress (*How can I assess whether I have achieved my learning goals?*)
3. Set learning goals (*Where do I see a need for improvement?*)
4. Design learning strategies (*What is the best way to learn the desired competency?*)
5. Consider each of the factors that influences learning, including metacognitive skills, executive functioning and self-regulation (*What will support or impede my learning?*)
6. Plan, implement and monitor learning progress (*How do I make sure that I stay focused and on track?*)
7. Evaluate your learning progress and metacognitive strategies (*How can I determine whether my learning strategies are effective?*)
8. Transfer what you have learned to new contexts, or to increasingly complex situations (*How can I extend the utility of my new skills?*)

Let us take a look at what you can do to address key items of your personalized metacognitive learning program.

Establishing a Mentalization Competency Baseline

In order to establish a baseline, you need to start with an assessment of your declarative knowledge, examining what you already know about mentalization and your mentalization strengths and weaknesses. At the same time, it is instructive to consider your metacognitive learning style, and your executive and self-regulatory functioning. The insights that you gain through these assessments should be tied to your baseline data and learning goals. Additionally, your understanding of what good mentalizing entails helps you select the criteria upon which you can judge your mentalization mastery. It is important to start with an assessment of your awareness and insight at each mentalization level. We begin with basic mentalizing.

ASSESSING BASIC MENTALIZING COMPETENCE

Basic mentalizing, as previously discussed, is critical to: detecting the nonverbal signals and cues that are necessary to make mental state inferences; connecting with others through nonverbal behavior, building rapport, and creating a positive ambiance so that people feel safe to share verbal and nonverbal behavior; being aware of our own susceptibility to "catching" the affective states of others, or to mimic their behavior; using these social information sources for mental state inferences; dissociating from others if we regard this type of sharing as unwelcome; and, being aware of interoceptive and exteroceptive sensations that can subconsciously influence us, and can bias our mental state inferences.

As part of your comprehensive self-assessment, you need to construct a basic mentalizing self-profile by:

1. Examining your understanding of embodied sharing of affect and behavior, and assessing your susceptibility to mimicry, affective contagion and behavioral contagion.
2. Establishing a baseline with regard to your nonverbal behavior encoding and decoding strengths and weaknesses.
3. Examining your awareness of interoceptive and exteroceptive stimuli, and assessing your ability to accurately attribute these sensations to their causes.

ASSESSING AFFECTIVE MENTALIZING COMPETENCE

Mentalizing at the affective level enables us to monitor the affective aspects of our interactions with others, to stay in conversational flow, and to keep our mentalization faculties online. Good affective mentalizing helps us to guard against fight, flight, or freeze reactions. It also helps us to maintain healthy relationships, and to restore good relations through empathizing, compassion and suitable affective communication.

Therefore, as part of your comprehensive self-assessment, you need to construct an affective mentalizing self-profile by:

1. Gauging your general understanding of affective mental states.
2. Exploring your attitude toward dealing with affective mental states of yourself and others.
3. Assessing the affective mental states and emotional styles with which you are comfortable/uncomfortable.
4. Examining your inclination toward affective and cognitive empathy.
5. Gauging your level of empathic distress.
6. Identifying the affect-regulation strategies that help you mitigate unhealthy levels of empathic distress.
7. Exploring your capacity for both self-focused and other-focused compassion.
8. Gauging your skills for affective explaining, affective message sending, and affective message receiving.

ASSESSING STRATEGIC MENTALIZING COMPETENCE

The final level, our highest and most cognitive level, of mentalization, strategic mentalizing, enables us to look beyond observable signals and cues to form increasingly rational models of what is going on in the minds of others, and in our own mind. Strategic mentalizing is used to infer intentions, attitudes, or motivations, in order to predict or explain complex goal-directed behavior, as well as people's orientations either to affiliate and cooperate with us (or others), or to socially distance from or compete against us (or others).

As part of your comprehensive self-assessment, you need to create a strategic mentalizing self-profile by:

1. Examining your motivation to strategically mentalize about others.
2. Exploring your ability to detect content in narratives and self-disclosures that has predictive and explanatory value.
3. Gauging your communication skills, in particular with regard to eliciting and facilitating narrative sharing and self-disclosure.
4. Examining the cognitive strategies that help you achieve accurate predictions and explanations of behavior.
5. Gauging the exercise of your influential power.
6. Examining your capacity for recognizing and resisting the unhealthy influence of others.

Inventories designed to assess the above-mentioned competencies are available at www.appliedtom.com.

DETERMINE YOUR POSITION ON SIX MENTALIZATION DIMENSIONS

Armed with the results of your comprehensive self-assessments you can determine your position on the spectra of the six mentalization dimensions, which were described in section I of this book:

1. "**Cognitivity**," ranging from *intuitive* to *reasoned* mentalizing.
2. "**Indicator focus**," ranging from *observed external* to *inferred internal* mentalizing.
3. "**Mental state focus**," ranging from *affective focused* to *cognitive focused* mentalizing.
4. "**Person focus**," ranging from *self-focused* to *other-focused* mentalizing.
5. "**Effort balance**," ranging from *hypermentalizing* to *hypomentalizing* mentalizing.
6. "**Mentalizing orientation**," ranging from an *affiliate/cooperate* to *socially distance/compete* mentalizing motivation.

ASSESSING COGNITIVE CONTROL AND FLEXIBILITY

Mentalization abilities are strongly associated with both executive functioning and self-regulation. We have divided the components of executive functioning and self-regulation into two categories: 1) those that are essential for cognitive control, and 2) those that are essential for cognitive flexibility. It is instructive to examine these abilities with regard to:

- "**Attention**" - critical to facilitating the focusing and monitoring of our activities and actions, and to alternating attention between others, ourselves and our surroundings, so as to gather relevant information required for mentalizing (perspective taking and gaining).
- "**Working memory**" - essential to integrating the information that we gather, associating the information with what we already know, and keeping in mind and contrasting different perspectives, strategies and concepts (perspective shifting).
- "**Prepotent response inhibition**" - critical to selecting the metacognitive and mentalization strategies that are more suitable than habitual reactions (impulse-regulation).
- "**Stress tolerance and management**" - important to balancing our affective reactions in order to keep metacognitive and mentalization faculties online and maintain conversational flow (affect-regulation).
- "**Goal-directedness**" - essential to meeting our metacognitive learning goals and our mentalization objectives (affiliation/cooperation or social distancing/competition).
- "**Metacognitive practices**" - critical to theory of mind reasoning and to understanding and enhancing our own metacognitive learning style (mentalization mastery).

Inventories designed to help you assess cognitive control and flexibility in relation to mentalization are available at www.appliedtom.com.

ASSESSING PERSONAL FACTORS

Additionally, it is beneficial to assess personal factors that can advance or impede your mentalization abilities, including:

- "**Temperament**" - hereditary factors that either promote or hinder the development of mentalization competencies. For instance, a person with a choleric temperament (mercurial, short-tempered and irritable) might find it difficult to stay calm and take the time necessary to gain another person's perspective.
- "**Personality traits**" - stable characteristics that describe or determine our mentalizing behavior across a spectrum of situations. Our personality traits are brought about by the dynamic interplay between our temperament and the sociocultural context of our upbringing and experiences in life.
- Other "**psychological**" or "**physiological characteristics**" that can promote or impede development of our mentalization abilities, such as alexithymia or autism.

ASSESSING ATTACHMENT STYLE

Attachment style is another assessable variable that can impact your motivation to mentalize and your mentalizing behavior. By way of review, four attachment styles have been identified:

1. "**Secure**" **attachment style**, characterized by a positive view of the self, others, and relationships, and by well-developed mentalization competencies.
2. "**Insecure-avoidant**" **attachment style**, characterized by a view of oneself as self-sufficient and without a need for, or interest in, close relationships. Individuals with this attachment style tend to avoid interacting with others, and often show a lack of interest in what is going on in the minds of other people.
3. "**Insecure-anxious**" **attachment style**, characterized by a negative view of oneself and a positive view of others. Individuals with this attachment style often mentalize for the need to control others and/or to control the situation. Moreover, such individuals have a hard time turning off higher-level mentalizing, even when it's not

required. Their mental state inferences are often strongly biased due to their anxious nature.

4. **"Insecure-disorganized" attachment style**, characterized by an alternating avoidant and anxious attachment behavioral style. These individuals tend to have an unstable and fluctuating and/or confused view of themselves and of others. Individuals with disorganized attachment style experience large fluctuations in their mentalizing motivation and accuracy due to a relentless internal conflict between wanting to be independent, while at the same time, having a strong need for dependency.

Indicia of Well-Developed Mentalization Competence

We have presented multiple avenues for assessing your mentalization strengths and weaknesses. The next step in the process is using this self-knowledge to design a metacognitive learning program aimed at enhancing your mentalization skills. This requires establishing criteria by which you can evaluate your learning progress. The following indicia of well-developed mentalization will help shape the criteria upon which you can judge the effectiveness of your learning program. A person with well-developed mentalization competencies:

- Demonstrates appreciation of both affective and cognitive mental states, including the interrelatedness of these states.
- Evinces an understanding that mental states are influenced by the backgrounds and personalities of people, by context and environment, and by interactions with others.
- Applies mentalization efforts guided by the premise that, in general, the complex mental states of others can be inferred only indirectly.

- Recognizes the margin of error of predictions and explanations of behavior based on mental state inferences.
- Acknowledges that mental states are mutable.
- Exhibits an appreciation of the fact that mental states of others often differ from their own mental states, but views these differences as an opportunity for investigation rather than a cause for discomfort.
- Demonstrates the ability to maintain, alternate and contrast different mental states and perspectives.
- Shows an appreciation of the fact that mental states can be confusing, and applies or elicits self-disclosure to clarify ambiguity, while employing appropriate self-regulation techniques.
- Validates mentalization challenges of others, and offers to help others gain an accurate understanding of mental states.
- Explains personal mental states, experiences, perspectives and intentions in a rich, clear and concise manner.
- Navigates flexibly between elementary, intuitive mentalizing and more effortful, high-level mentalizing, adjusting and balancing mentalization activities to meet situational demands.
- Alternates appropriately between *intra*personal, *inter*personal and *extra*personal mentalizing.
- Displays a keen awareness of both verbal and nonverbal signals and cues.
- Demonstrates attentive mentalizing readiness, as appropriate, in light of the circumstances.
- Explains affective mental states in a rich, clear and concise manner, and sends and receives affective messages appropriately.
- Acknowledges changes in affective mental states, and employs affect regulation skills to keep emotions from becoming disruptive.
- Demonstrates mentalization efforts aimed at increasing affiliation and cooperation as required by the situation.
- Demonstrates competitive or social distancing mentalization efforts as required by the situation.

- Displays influential power, and selects appropriate influence tactics to shape the environment and to resist the unwanted influence of others.

From a more general point of view, a competent mentalizer:

- Demonstrates a genuine interest in the mental states and perspectives of others, free of any intention to use this social information to inappropriately exercise control over others.
- Exhibits a healthy psychological and sociological appreciation of mental processes.
- Remains at ease with, and open to, exploring uncomfortable topics and painful memories and experiences.
- Interprets mentalizing awareness and behavior from a metacognitive perspective.
- Demonstrates well-developed communication skills and applies these skills in a relaxed manner that invites narrative sharing and self-disclosure.
- Displays empathy and compassion in a timely and appropriate fashion.
- Narrates experiences and self-disclosures in a rich and coherent manner that demonstrates autobiographical continuity.
- Acknowledges misunderstandings and miscommunication and takes corrective action in a calm and constructive way.
- Accepts responsibility for, takes ownership of, and corrects personal behavior that disrupts the flow of interactions with others.
- Understands how interoceptive and exteroceptive sensations can impact perceptions.
- Demonstrates a sympathetic and forgiving attitude when dealing with conflict and misunderstanding.

Recognizing Poor Mentalization Competence

Part of learning to be a good mentalizer involves learning how to recognize poor mentalizing in yourself and in others. Having well-developed mentalization skills yourself does not guarantee successful interactions with others, especially those who are struggling with severely underdeveloped mentalization skills. A person with underdeveloped mentalization competencies:

- Demonstrates a social reasoning approach that is devoid of mental state references.
- Displays a lack of interest in mental states, possibly showing signs of defensiveness, denial, irritation, or aggression when faced with mental state inquiries.
- Employs a rigid mentalization style, approaching experiences, mental states, or perspectives from a black or white, all or nothing, good or bad, right or wrong perspective.
- Shows a strong certainty about mental state inferences, predictions and explanations without sufficient evidentiary support.
- Tends to ignore the knowledge states of others, focusing instead on extraneous details, and ignoring relevant facts.
- Displays a one-dimensional interest in mental states, either self-directed or other-directed.
- Demonstrates a disproportionately strong focus on instrumental goals, while ignoring relational goals during interactions with others.
- Explains social interactions from an exclusively intuitive or analytical perspective.
- Demonstrates a strong focus on certain mental states, while ignoring other more relevant mental states.
- Mentalizes in a generalized, biased, or stereotypical way, showing a lack of attributional complexity.

- Relies exclusively on internal aspects (desires, beliefs) or on external aspects (facial expressions, tone of voice) of others, failing to take into account consistencies or inconsistencies between the two different vectors.
- Explains intentions and motivations of others without consideration of context, or based upon the unsubstantiated assumption that intentions and motivations of others are ill-intended.
- Automatically looks for others to blame when things go wrong.
- Attributes behavior to personality, rather than situational causes.
- Demonstrates a lack of insight regarding the impact that a person's behavior has on others.

From a more general point of view, a person with underdeveloped mentalization competencies:

- Demonstrates a lack of the healthy and appropriate influential power needed to reach personal objectives (without taking advantage of, or being taken advantage by, others).
- Displays a superficial or hyper intellectualized narrative/self-disclosure style.
- Exhibits underdeveloped communication skills (e.g., poor listening skills), often owing to an absence of interest in the mental states or perspectives of others.
- Applies an authoritarian or condescending communication style that discourages others from self-disclosure or narrative sharing.
- Fails to detect and repair misunderstandings and communications that have gone off track.

Bateman and Fonagy describe in their book Mentalization-Based Treatment for Personality Disorders: A Practical Guide (2016) three dominant methods of non-mentalizing, which they refer to as pre-mentalization modes, consisting of:

1. "**Teleological thinking**," which involves making mental state assumptions on the basis of a person's actions without any effort to gain the perspective of the actor. For instance, "She didn't greet me while she was driving by; therefore, she is avoiding me."
2. "**Psychic equivalence**," a form of projection in which one's own internal mental states are equated with the mental states of others. This mode blocks all curiosity about alternative perspectives of others. An example of psychic equivalence would be concluding that someone else is angry because that reflects your own current mental state.
3. "**Pretend mode**," involves a mental state in which the mental world is poorly connected with the external reality. In this pre-mentalization mode a person's thoughts and feelings, or the descriptions of other people's mental states, are overly elaborate, loosely connected to what really happened, and not based on evidence.

The failure to mentalize accurately (or the failure to mentalize at all) is often due to developmental deficiency or psychophysiological conditions. Nevertheless, everyone struggles at times with mentalization, especially in stressful situations and unfamiliar environments.

Recognizing Pseudomentalization

As we have seen, there are those who use a "factitious" form of mentalization, coined by Bateman and Fonagy (2016) as pseudomentalization, as a means of manipulating and controlling others. The objective of pseudomentalization is to bring about confusion and frustration in others. Bateman and Fonagy explain that "[p]seudomentalizing can occur exclusively in specific relations, for instance, with a certain caregiver with whom the person has an unhealthy attachment relationship. It can also occur exclusively in a particular context that a person finds stressful." As Bateman and Fonagy point out, however, it can be attributed to underdeveloped mentalization skills or other impairment. Bateman and Fonagy (2016) described four pseudomentalizing subtypes that may be observed in people, especially those who suffer from a personality disorder such as borderline personality disorder or narcissism:

1. "**Intrusive mentalizing**," which is characterized by a tendency to intrude on and manipulate other people's life through reflections of one's inner world that do not seem to be genuine. In section II of this book, we described a pseudomentalization tactic known as cold reading, a ploy whereby the so-called "mentalist" implies that he knows much more about the subject than he actually does. This kind of pseudomentalizing is often experienced by a subject as intrusive, disconcerting, or annoying. As Bateman and Fonagy propose, this kind of pseudomentalizing can be effectively counteracted by challenging the assumptions of the mentalizer.
2. "**Overactive-inaccurate mentalizing**," which entails a preoccupation with mental states, often looking for signals and cues that might reveal something negative about the person who is being mentalized or about the situation. People who engage in this subtype of pseudomentalization often see meaning in nonverbal and verbal behavior that would be interpreted as neutral by others. Their interpretation of the social information they gather is often inappropriate and without a genuine interest in true mental states.
3. "**Destructively inaccurate mentalizing**," which involves an extreme projection of the "mentalizer's" own feelings and thoughts onto others, for instance by asserting "*You were asking me to hit you*," or "*You are trying to drive me crazy*." Convinced with the unassailability of his own inferences, the "mentalizer" simply proceeds to act in accordance with his assumptions, leaving no room for the other person to set the record straight. The best way to deal with this kind of pseudomentalizing is to withdraw from the interaction and revisit

the event at a later time when things have settled down. This will provide you with a better opportunity to understand and explain your true feelings and thoughts.

4. "**Bizarre mentalizing**," which is characterized by highly inaccurate mental state attributions and mental state inferences that are completely disconnected from reality or even implausible psychologically.

Pseudomentalization tactics can leave us feeling as though the "mentalizer" is trying to manipulate or control us (which is often the case). At a minimum, we can interpret pseudomentalization as an attempt to provoke us, eliciting anxiety or anger. It registers as an assault on our sense of self, our self-confidence and our self-identity.

Pseudomentalization is often used by people with antisocial personality disorder to provoke anger or fear. People with a narcissistic personality tend to revert to pseudomentalizing when they feel entitled, when their position is challenged, or when their ego is threatened. This form of pseudomentalization is purely self-serving.

Pseudomentalizing behavior can also be seen in people with borderline personality disorder (BPD), who use these tactics on account of their insecurities with unstable relationships, their fragile sense of self, and their emotional volatility. As discussed in previous chapters, BPD individuals are identifiable by their inaccurate, or absence of, self-mentalizing. They do tend to understand their own desires and knowledge states well, however.

Once you have a clear understanding of your mentalization strengths and weaknesses and have established a baseline to measure your learning progress, you can select appropriate learning goals, and describe the benchmarks against which you can judge the quality of your mentalizing.

Designing Strategies to Master Mentalization

Let us examine what you can do to satisfy steps three, four and five of the metacognitive learning sequence:

3. Set learning goals (*Where do I see a need for improvement?*)
4. Design learning strategies (*What is the best way to learn or improve my mentalization competency?*)
5. Consider each of the factors that influences learning, including metacognitive skills, executive functioning and self-regulation (*What will support or impede my learning progress?*)

Your learning strategies need to be attached to the learning goals that are based upon the insights you have gained from your self-assessment. With regard to basic mentalizing, for instance, a learning goal could be to gain a deeper understanding of, and broader experience with, the embodied sharing of affect and behavior. A related goal might be to enhance your ability to detect relevant embodied signals and cues.

An additional learning objective could be to strengthen your detection acuity and decoding proficiency in dealing with nonverbal behavior, with the aim of becoming more mindful of the various channels through which people communicate nonverbally. You might also want to consider the goal of sharpening your nonverbal encoding skills to increase appropriate and effective use of the same nonverbal communication channels. Because the capacity for attentional control and flexibility is critical to detecting and decoding nonverbal indicators, an additional learning objective could be to enhance your attentional direction and focus.

Another learning goal could be to improve your detection and interpretation of intero- and exteroceptive stimuli (your body awareness), in order to facilitate a more volitional, "top down" approach, as opposed to a reactive "bottom up" approach.

With regard to affective mentalizing, a learning goal might be to broaden your understanding of, and familiarity with, affective mental states.

Additionally, you could choose the goal of deepening your understanding of affective and cognitive empathy practices in order to achieve a comprehensive and accurate understanding of the affective states and needs of others.

A related goal could be to learn how to minimize empathic distress through enhancement of your affect regulation skills, the mental processes that come into play in attending to, selecting and successfully monitoring and controlling thoughts, emotions and behaviors.

Strengthening your compassionate skills is another useful goal to consider. While empathy training focuses on the detection and understanding of the suffering of others, compassion training focuses on the alleviation of this suffering. Your capacity for compassion can be enhanced on two levels: compassion for others and self-compassion.

With regard to affective communication, you might include objectives aimed at sharpening the clarity of your affective self-disclosures and affective message sending, and refining your affective message receptivity skills.

With regard to strategic mentalizing, a critical learning objective could be to reinforce constructive motivations and cultivate a healthy motivational balance. This can be achieved, in part, through enhancing your understanding of the elements of strategic mentalizing. A constituent goal could be to enhance your ability to extract from narratives and self-disclosures the type of content that has predictive and explanatory value, and to understand how to assess the validity of this content. A closely related objective could be to strengthen your ability to associate extracted content with primary mental states, such as beliefs and knowledge, and with the more complex mental states of intention, motivation and attitude.

An additional learning goal you might want to include is improving your understanding of how basic mentalizing and affective mentalizing can facilitate and inform your theory of mind.

Another training objective could be to increase your flexibility in employing perspective taking, gaining, shifting and shaping in your theory of mind reasoning. Along similar lines, you could consider adding the goal of deepening your understanding of, and experience with, the critical thinking skills and methodologies that are essential for theory of mind reasoning, such as attributional complexity, analytical thinking and metacognitive thinking.

You might also want to devote time and effort to enhancement of the adaptable communication skills that promote perspective sharing and insight.

Finally, your learning trajectory could include goals aimed at improving your influential power to persuade others and to resist the unwanted influence of others.

FOCUSED MENTALIZING LEARNING GOALS

In addition to these general learning goals, you might want to consider more focused learning goals aimed at improving your ability to mentalize more accurately when dealing with people who have psychological impairments, or are struggling with personality disorders. Another specialized training area to consider could be cross-cultural mentalizing. Training objectives could also be directed at enhancing your level of cognitive control and cognitive flexibility, as both of these faculties enhance strategic mentalizing indirectly.

Once you have established your potential learning needs and selected your learning goals, you need to consider factors that could facilitate or impede your learning progress.

Finally, you are ready to plan and implement your learning trajectory and monitor your learning progress.

Linear, Cyclical and Holistic Learning

This brings us to the final three steps of the metacognitive learning sequence:

6. Plan, implement and monitor your learning progress (*How do I make sure that I stay focused and on track?*)
7. Evaluate your learning progress and metacognitive strategies (*How can I determine whether my learning strategies are effective?*)
8. Transfer what you have learned to new contexts or to increasingly complex situations (*How can I extend the utility of my new skills?*)

Your metacognitive learning program should incorporate linear, cyclical and holistic learning models. A linear learning model progresses from one step to the next, and requires that you follow a learning sequence from beginning to end. Generally, a linear model for learning mentalization competencies should contain the following sequential steps:

1. Expand your declarative knowledge with regard to the competency you want to strengthen, for instance, by reading books, by researching information on the internet, or by consulting experts.
2. Explore possible learning strategies and select the most suitable strategies to fit your learning goals and your learning style.
3. Design your learning plan, including a visualization of your learning trajectory, to provide you with guidance and help you stay on track.
4. Gather and organize resources that you need.
5. Plan for the learning activities (time, place, people, etc.).
6. Implement the plan and monitor your progress.

A cyclical learning model involves repetition and refinement of a sequential learning model. In each iteration, you assess your success in learning and applying new cognitive, affective and behavioral skills; you determine how effective your learning strategies are; and you gauge how well you have achieved your specific learning objectives. You need to practice, evaluate, adjust and repeat this cycle until your new mentalization skills become second nature and, consequently, less effortful.

The holistic model guides your integration of all the different competencies you have learned, and your generalization of these competencies across different social contexts. It is at this level of your learning trajectory that you truly achieve mastery of mentalization, which means that:

- You have developed an automated, intuitive and generalized mentalization understanding and practice.
- Your mentalization activities have become more second nature and less effortful, while your predictions and explanations of human behavior have become increasingly accurate.
- Your mentalization competencies are well supported by enhanced skills, mental faculties and behaviors that facilitate mentalization (i.e., cognitive control and flexibility, verbal and nonverbal communication, empathy and compassion).
- You can flexibly migrate between lower and higher levels of mentalization in line with contextual demands.
- You can achieve a healthy balance on each of the six mentalization dimensions in congruence with contextual demands.

Each learning assignment needs to be developed in such a way that it stimulates different sensorial modes (information channels). Additionally, your assignments should incorporate intra-, inter- and extrapersonal learning settings. The more information channels you use, and the wider the variety of practice settings, the better able you will be to generalize your learning to fit a holistic framework.

Some people have a strong preference for using one particular sensorial channel or context to learn new skills. Such preferences are indicative of your personal learning style. To a certain extent, it is wise to align your learning exercises with your preferred learning style, as it will make your learning efforts feel more natural. We strongly recommend, however, that you also incorporate less familiar, but equally suitable, learning strategies, as this will broaden your comfort zone and expand your learning opportunities significantly. Let us take a look at the different information channels and practice settings that are available:

- "**Visual**" - learning through observation, for instance, by watching other people in social situations.
- "**Aural**" - learning through listening, for instance, by focusing on the verbal and nonverbal auditory reactions of others, or listening to the way experts handle social situations.
- "**Verbal**" - learning by asking yourself and others questions about your skills and about how others perform similar skills.
- "**Physical**" - experiential learning whereby you practice your skills in real-time social contexts.
- "**Logical**" - cognitive learning through logical reasoning, for instance, by using attributional complexity.
- "**Solitary**" (intrapersonal learning) - for instance, by exploring theoretical concepts to improve your subject matter expertise.
- "**Social**" (interpersonal learning) - for instance, by practicing your skills within concrete social settings.
- "**Contextual**" and "**situational**" (extrapersonal learning) - for instance, by practicing new skills in different sociocultural settings, or by using interactions that are mediated by social media platforms.

In conclusion, metacognitive learning is a powerful educational tool that can be employed to:

- Broaden your repertoire of strategies and meta-strategies that help you to learn new mentalization skills.
- Gain metacognitive insight into why, when and where to use these strategies.
- Acquire knowledge of the tactics used in support of these strategies.
- Develop automaticity and flexibility in applying what you have learned.

Well-developed mentalization competencies will strengthen your social intuition, which will guide your interactions with others and enable you to make healthy social decisions quickly and efficiently.

Nine Mentalization Maxims

This brings us to the end of this final chapter on mastering mentalization. As you design and implement your personalized learning trajectory, remain mindful of the benefits of accurate and appropriate mentalizing as embodied in our nine mentalization maxims:

1. *Understand others* and you will **be appreciated**.
2. *Assert yourself duly* and you will **be respected**.
3. *Be open to critique* and you will **gain insight**.
4. *Display prosocial behavior* and you will **find cooperation**.
5. *Show competence and sound moral conduct* and you will **be trusted**.
6. *Communicate with Grice's maxims in mind* and you will **be understood**.
7. *Cooperate aptly with others* and you will **be valued**.
8. *Compete with integrity* and you will **find generosity**.
9. *Interact with compassion* and you will **be seen as humane**.

References

Bateman, A & Fonagy P. (2016). *Mentalization-Based Treatment for Personality Disorders: A Practical Guide*. Oxford University Press.

Kuhn, D. (2000). *Theory of mind, metacognition, and reasoning: A life-span perspective.* In P. Mitchell & K. J. Riggs (Eds.), *Children's reasoning and the mind* (p. 301–326). Psychology Press/Taylor & Francis (UK).

Schraw, G., & Dennison, R. S. (1994). Assessing Metacognitive Awareness. *Contemporary Educational Psychology, 19*(4), 460–475. doi:10.1006/ceps.1994.1033

Index

E

F

G

H

I

J

K

L

M

N

O

P

T

V

W

Y

www.appliedtom.com

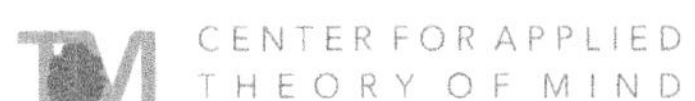

Made in the USA
Las Vegas, NV
23 October 2024

10338809R00201